D0290354

KATHY SMITH'S WALKFIT™ FOR A BETTER BODY is. . .

- A perfect path to fitness, total body toning, fat burning, weight control, stress reduction, and improved cardiovascular health.
- Safe and effective. So easy on your body, there's rarely a reason not to do it.
- Adjustable. Pick your own pace from moderate activity to high-intensity workout.
- Light on your heavy schedule and easy on your budget.
- A self-esteem builder—no matter what shape you're in, it's a program that will lift your spirits and improve your health from day one.
- Convenient. Do it anytime, anywhere.

Optimum health isn't a myth or a dream. It's simple. It's easy. And it's within walking distance!

KATHY SMITH is a longtime leader in the fitness industry. She has reached millions of people with information on health, fitness, and nutrition. Kathy is the creator of 15 fitness videos that have topped the *Billboard* bestseller charts for more than 10 years. She is the national spokesperson and development team member for Reebok's Body Walk program. Her involvement with non-profit organizations includes spokesperson for the National Recreation and Parks Association as well as Allstate Insurance's "Just Say Go," a fitness program designed for elementary schools. She is a veteran fitness correspondent of NBC's *Today* show, ABC's *Good Morning America*, and Whittle Communications' *Special Reports TV*. Her Pregnancy Workout was praised by the American Film Institute, the National Education Association, and *Billboard* magazine. She serves on the board of directors of ECO, the Earth Communications Office, and The Women's Sports Foundation. She lives with her husband and two daughters in California.

SUSANNA LEVIN is a contributing editor for *Walking* magazine, and her articles on health have appeared in *Self, Outside, American Health, Fitness, New Choices, Shape, Essence, Men's Fitness, The Physician and Sportsmedicine*, and other magazines.

KATHY SMITH'S

WALKFIT™
FOR A
BETTER BODY

KATHY SMITH
with Susanna Levin

WARNER BOOKS

A Time Warner Company

Before beginning this or any other exercise or nutritional
regimen, consult your physician to be sure it is appropriate for you.
The information in this book reflects the author's experiences
and is not intended to replace medical advice. Any questions
regarding your individual health, general or specific, should be
addressed to your physician.

Copyright © 1994 by Kathy Smith Enterprises, Inc.
All rights reserved.

Warner Books, Inc., 1271 Avenue of the Americas, New York, NY 10020

 A Time Warner Company

Printed in the United States of America

ISBN 0-446-67048-0

Cover design by Diane Luger

Photography by Mark Hanauer

Book design by Giorgetta Bell McRee

Acknowledgments

I would like to thank my husband, Steve Grace, who's been a willing convert to the fitness lifestyle. Steve's contribution to this book included walking 11-minute miles, reading chapters until one in the morning, and consistently producing keen insights. His understanding of my philosophy—and his vocal enthusiasm for the virtues of counting fat grams—were invaluable. Most of all, Steve kept everybody laughing, even as deadlines piled up around us.

Thanks also to Reebok, for their continuing support both for me and for walking. Reebok's commitment to developing great shoes and educating walking instructors across the United States is bringing the joys of walking to more people.

Without the efforts of Russ Kamalski, Joanne Feldman, and the entire team in the office, none of this would have been possible. They make my life and my business work, which gives me time to put my creative energy into other projects.

Betsy Horton LaForge helped bring sense and sanity to the confusion over diet and nutrition. Leslie Pam, Ph.D., provided great insight into motivation. Nicky Evans applied her boundless energies to bringing the WALKFIT program together. Nicky is New Zealand's greatest export. Thanks also to Felicia Eth, and Nanscy Neiman and Joann Davis of Warner Books.

Walking Magazine has supported the efforts of both authors, and its editorial staff provides walkers everywhere with a lively, intelligent, and reliable source for information.

Finally, great thanks to Don and Sharon Schiltz of Bigfork, Montana. This book was hatched in their guest room on the very same day the wild turkey chicks were hatched in the shed.

Contents

KATHY SMITH'S
WALKFIT™
— FOR A —
BETTER BODY

1

The Walk of Life

This book came to life, naturally enough, on a walk. It was August, and I was in Bigfork, Montana, on a much-needed summer vacation with my husband, Steve, and our daughters, Katie, who was four years old, and Perrie, who was two. My coauthor, Sue Levin, came up for a visit, and on a bright, cloudless Monday morning, Sue and I left the girls with Steve and headed off to nearby Big Mountain for a walk.

In the course of planning this book, I'd spoken to Sue on the phone many times, but we'd never met in person. A walk seemed the ideal way to get better acquainted. The trail I chose for us to walk wound from the bottom of Big Mountain to the top, about 5 miles in all, through the Flathead National Forest. We found the trailhead and set out at a quick tempo. Soon we were into the rhythm of the walk, working up a sweat.

We were breathing hard in the thin mountain air, but not so hard that we couldn't talk. We started out sharing our ideas for the book, but the conversation soon turned to more personal subjects: family, friendships, relationships, and kids. That's not such a big leap, really, because walking is something I associate with family and friends.

In fact, I first got into walking five years ago, when I was pregnant with Katie. In about the fifth month, Steve and I started taking long walks in the evening. It was a wonderful way to be together, to get into one another's thoughts, and to imagine the ways in which our life was about to change.

The habit lasted well beyond that pregnancy, and walking is now a vital part of my life. Walking workouts are a regular part of my training, and walking is an important family activity for us, as well. Steve and I love to hike and walk together, and we regularly take the girls on walks around the neighborhood or on "adventure hikes" in the nearby state parks.

On that August morning in Montana, Sue and I walked and talked for close to two hours, stopping only to take swigs of water or admire the Rocky Mountain wildflowers—mariposa lily, Indian paintbrush, penstemon, and Montana bear grass. The western Montana landscape was inspirational, with the jagged, granite peaks of Glacier Park off in the distance, and ideas seemed to come one after another. By the time we reached the top of the mountain, I felt as if the book was all but finished.

As I walked around town later that day, I was especially conscious of how good I felt. My legs were loose and light, and my whole body felt flexible and centered. I felt energized, as if walking had charged some battery deep inside.

After that walk, this book seemed more important than ever. I was reminded of just how much walking has done for me in the last five years. I won't kid you—the fat-burning and cardiovascular conditioning benefits are important to me. We walked fast, and that's crucial for a high-intensity workout. (We'll talk a lot in this book about techniques for increasing walking speed, so you can get more from your walks.) But even at that fast pace, I enjoyed myself every step of the way and felt great afterward.

I want more people to see for themselves that there *is* an exercise that accomplishes your physical goals—increased fitness and cardiovascular health, muscle toning, and weight management—while it feeds your soul. Forty minutes of fast walking will strengthen your heart, lungs, and muscles, and burn calories as well, but it can also be much more than that. It's time for talking, time for thinking. It's time to do for yourself what needs to be done.

A LIFELONG ACTIVITY

I wish I had a nickel for every time I've heard someone say that walking is a "lifelong activity." When people use that expression, what they usually mean is that walking is a good exercise for when you're old, and that's a mistake that needs to be corrected. Walking is a great workout for *anyone*, at any age.

Walking *is* ideal for older people, but it's also ideal for young people, highly fit people, people who need to lose weight, and everyone in between. There are two big reasons why walking does so much for so many.

First, walking is so simple, so convenient, and so easy on your bones and joints that there's never a reason *not* to do it: It's the "no-excuse" workout. That means it's easier to be consistent about exercise, and consistency is the real key to lifelong health and fitness. Consistency doesn't mean "being good" for weeks or even months. It means finding ways to make exercise a regular part of your life.

Second, walking is as hard as you make it. Depending

on your pace, walking can be either a moderate activity (3 to 4 MPH) or a high-intensity workout (4 to 5 MPH). The fitter you are, the faster you have to walk for cardiovascular conditioning benefits, but *anyone*, no matter how fit, can get a workout from walking.

With WALKFIT®, you'll learn techniques for fast walking: changes in your stride that can really get you cranking. The cardiovascular and calorie demands of walking fast are as high—if not higher—than those that come with any kind of aerobic exercise: At 5 MPH, you can burn 9 calories per minute or more. That's close to 600 calories per hour!

Together, consistency and speed form the basis of my walking program. The short-term goal is to get you walking four to six times per week at a pace that's fast enough to get the results you want, but not so fast that you don't enjoy yourself. That's because the long-term goal is to get you hooked on a lifelong habit of regular, fast walking.

CONSISTENCY

It's becoming increasingly clear from research into exercise that the greatest health benefits come from regular, moderate exercise. When researchers look at how lifestyle affects health, they find a huge difference between the inactive person and the regularly active person. There's less of a difference between the regularly active person and the super-fit person.

In other words, the greatest gains come when you go from doing nothing to doing something regularly. That's why consistency is so important.

If you're trying to lose weight and keep it off, consistency is the difference between success and failure. Research into weight loss overwhelmingly shows that unless you make *regular* exercise a part of your life, you're fighting an uphill battle. One recent study comparing "regainers" and "maintainers" in a weight-loss program provided dramatic proof of this: Of the maintainers (those who kept the weight off), 90 percent exercised regularly, compared to only 34 percent of the regainers.

If reading this book is a step toward getting consistent about exercise, you're making a healthy choice. Even if you're a "non-fitness-oriented" person (a politically correct alternative for "couch potato" that I just made up), and even if other tries at getting in shape haven't worked for you, the odds are very high that you can succeed with walking. Why? Because walking is easier to stick with than other forms of exercise.

I think lots of people have the same experience as Joy Montarbo, a 35-year-old mother of five from Vancouver, Washington. I went for a walk with Joy during a WALKFIT promotion in Portland, Oregon, and she told me that before she started WALKFIT, she tried all kinds of exercise programs but was never able to stick with them.

"I would try something, but then I'd get bored or have too much work, so I stopped," she said. She started WALK-FIT as part of a weight-loss program, and now she's been at it for almost two years, walking four 13-minute miles, five days a week.

To Joy, the difference is plain to see: "When exercise is hard, it's easier *not* to do it. But walking is so easy—you don't need anything except your shoes. Walking is an escape for me. It's time to get away from the kids and do my own thing."

THE NO-EXCUSE WORKOUT

It's easy to understand why walking works so well when you consider the common reasons I hear for why people don't exercise:

"There's no room in my life for exercise." Some people simply have less time—or are less willing to invest a lot of time—in exercise. Then there are those days when you've only got a half-hour of breathing room from the moment you get up until your head hits the pillow again. Well, a half-hour to forty minutes is all you need for a walk. If you use that breathing room for some heavy breathing—on a day when you otherwise wouldn't have done anything—you're taking a big step toward consistency.

Walking doesn't have to make a big dent in your time budget. Your workout time is minimal, and there's no driving to and from the gym or the pool. In a pinch, you don't even have to change clothes or shower. Just put on your walking shoes, take a fast spin around the neighborhood, and pick up your day where you left off. Or walk to work, on errands, or out to dinner and the movies.

"I just don't have the energy to get started." While the idea of going for a run or doing an exercise class can seem overwhelming, a walk is a more manageable goal. It doesn't take a tremendous amount of motivation to get out the door for a walk, and after a few minutes your energy always seems to kick in.

Energy is like wealth: The rich get richer, and the energetic get more energy. The effort you invest in getting out the door is returned, with interest, by walking. You end up with more energy not only for exercise, but for the rest of life as well.

"I started an exercise class, but I didn't know what I was doing. I couldn't keep up, and I was exhausted after two weeks." When you're at the bottom of the learning curve looking up, it's easy to feel out of shape, out of step, and defeated. With walking, you got past the learning curve when you were about two feet tall. In this program, I'll add some new techniques to your stride, but it's nothing you can't master right away. So your walking workouts will feel good—and you'll get results—from day one.

"I always seem to get aches and pains after a few weeks, and by the time I get better, I've lost my motivation." It's extremely unlikely that you'll have to stop walking due to injury. But with all the emphasis on the fact that walking doesn't *hurt* your body, I think people often overlook how *good* walking makes your body feel. What I really love about a walking workout is that the muscles in my back, butt, abdominals, and hips all feel really loose and strong afterward.

NOT JUST FOR NOVICES

Strangely enough, it's often easier to talk non-exercisers into walking than it is to get fit people to give it a try. When these folks come down from their "I'm too fit for walking" high horse, they discover the training advantages of walking.

Chris Evert and I have been very good friends for a long time now. Recently Chris was in Los Angeles to play in a benefit tennis tournament. The day after her match, she came out with me for "a little walk." I set out at my normal 12-minute-mile pace (I actually slowed down a little for her sake), and Chris was stunned when she couldn't keep up with me. At the end of the walk, she was amazed by how hard she'd worked, and now she's a WALKFIT convert. (Of course, Chris got even with me a little while later when I went to visit her in Aspen, by taking me hiking at 9,000 feet. You should have seen her grin when I waved the white flag.)

The key for fit people is to find the walking pace that's fast enough to challenge your cardiovascular system. Then walking provides top-notch aerobic training—no ifs, ands, or buts about it. The easiest way to prove it is to get you to try walking 3 miles in 36 minutes. No matter how fit you are, you'll have to work hard to get to that pace and hold it.

Fast walking is also ideal for long, slow distance (LSD) training. LSD training, which elite athletes use to maximize their endurance, is a long workout—90 minutes or more—done at a relatively low intensity (around 65 percent of your maximum heart rate). If you usually run or do aerobics for 45 minutes, you don't get much LSD training. While it's neither practical nor appealing to do a two-hour run or two hours of aerobics, you *can* do a two-hour fast walk. This kind of sustained effort is also very good for fat burning.

Walking has the additional advantage of causing minimal wear-and-tear on bones and joints. If you've been active for a long time, especially if you've suffered from joint injuries in the past, now is the time to take remedial action. Switching to a lower-impact form of aerobic training while you're still in good shape is a great way to ensure that you stay that way.

For cross-training, walking has all the benefits I've mentioned and more. Alternating higher-impact activities like running or step aerobics with a couple of hard walks a week can make your body feel really good, without compromising your fitness gains. In fact, adding these high-aerobic, low-impact sessions can improve total fitness by allowing musculo-skeletal systems to recover, and by preventing overtraining injuries and burn-out.

Last year I was teaching fast-walking techniques at a Reebok-sponsored clinic at a Los Angeles health club. Diane Ekker, a friend of mine who is an aerobics instructor at the club, came to the clinic. A few months later, Diane mentioned to me that she had added fast walking to her weekly cross-training routine. Diane was doing 5 miles over a hilly route around her neighborhood in 60 minutes—that's a 12-minute-per-mile pace!

"The first few times, I was sore afterward—my butt, shoulders, and back, particularly, and that surprised me,"

Diane said. It's understandable that she didn't expect to be sore. In addition to teaching five aerobics classes a week, she's an excellent runner and lifts weights regularly. But walking taxed her muscles in new ways.

I asked Diane why she kept with it. "I like the cross-training benefits," she explained. "I used to run five times a week, and that's pretty stressful on your feet and joints. This lets me cut back on my running and still get a real good cardiovascular workout. I have to push myself, and when I'm done I really feel like I had a good workout."

SIMPLE, NOT EASY

Diane admitted to me that she'd been skeptical before the clinic. Because she's so very fit, she doubted that walking would be enough of a cardiovascular challenge for her. "When I went to the workshop, I thought, 'What are they going to do, teach us how to walk?' But they did," she said.

Like Diane, many people think that because walking is simple, it's also easy—i.e., not physically taxing. In fact, the single most important thing to keep in mind as you start this program is this: If walking is really going to work for you, you're really going to have to work at walking.

I don't mean to take anything away from going for a stroll. If you switch from doing nothing to strolling five days a week, you're taking a tremendous step toward good health. In fact, an important recent study from the Cooper Institute for Aerobic Research, published in the *Journal of the American Medical Association*, found that women between the ages of 20 and 40 who took a slow, 3-mile stroll five times per week increased their HDL, or "good" cholesterol, levels significantly, even though they weren't walking fast enough to improve their aerobic fitness. In other words, while these women didn't technically get fitter, they still got healthier.

But if your goal is aerobic fitness, muscle toning, and calorie burning for weight loss or weight control, you're going to have to do more than easy strolling. Think of it this way: Speed burns.

Here's why: Your body is comfortable at your normal walking pace because it's working very efficiently. But efficiency is your enemy: As with a fuel-efficient car, the most efficient pace burns the fewest calories. As soon as you walk faster than your normal "around town" pace, your body starts using more oxygen and burning calories at a higher rate. So to really maximize your walking workouts, you're going to have to sacrifice a little comfort.

The faster you walk, the more calories you burn. For example, at a pace of 20 minutes per mile (3 MPH), you burn about 3 calories per minute. At a 15-minute-mile pace (4 MPH), that goes up to 4 to 6 calories per minute. So by increasing your pace by 1 mile per hour, you can just about double your caloric expenditure. This effect gets even stronger when you can get your speed up to a very fast 12 minutes per mile (5 MPH), where you'll burn a phenomenal *9 calories per minute.*

If you walk for 45 minutes, five times a week, you'll burn 1,350 more calories at a 5-MPH pace than you would walking 3 MPH. Over the course of a year, that adds up to nearly 20 extra pounds of fat that you'll burn—just by speeding up!

These are average numbers of calories burned per hour for different walking speeds:

Pace	Calories burned in an hour
2.0 mph/30-minute miles	120 to 180
3.0 mph/20-minute miles	180 to 240
4.0 mph/15-minute miles	240 to 360
5.0 mph/12-minute miles	450 to 600

In general, the more you weigh, the more calories you'll burn. If you weigh more than 150 pounds, for example, you may burn even more calories than it says here. Caloric expenditure is also affected by *how* you walk: If you pump your arms or actively push off with your toes, for example, you'll burn more.

Of course, it's obviously true that the longer you walk, the more calories you burn. That's why some people say that for weight loss, it's best to walk slower, longer. But that assumes it's an either/or proposition: Either you walk fast and get tired quickly, or you walk slowly for a long time.

This program is about walking faster, longer. You're going to learn to modify your stride so that you can walk at higher speeds, thereby burning more calories for a longer time. The idea is not to walk so fast that you're exhausted after 15 minutes. This isn't race walking, but it sure ain't strolling, either!

MORE VOTES FOR SPEED

Speed does a lot more than burn calories. A faster pace takes your heart rate higher, which means greater gains for your heart, lungs, and circulatory system. In the study of women walkers I mentioned earlier, a second group of women walked at a 5-MPH pace (12 minutes per mile).

They had an average heart rate of 163 beats per minute, or 86 percent of their maximum, compared to the 3-MPH strollers, whose average heart rate was 106 (57 percent of maximum heart rate). A third group, who walked at 4 MPH (15-minute miles) got their heart rates up to 126 (67 percent of maximum heart rate).

After six weeks in this study, the 5-MPH walkers had increased their cardiovascular fitness, as measured by their maximum oxygen consumption, by 16 percent—four times as much as the strollers! The 4-MPH walkers improved twice as much as the strollers, but only half as much as the 5-MPH walkers.

That all boils down to this: The faster you walk, the fitter you're going to get, and if you walk *very* fast, you can get *very* fit.

When you walk faster, you also engage more muscles in your walking stride, and demand more of them, which results in conditioning and toning. You'll feel—and eventually see—that extra effort in your upper thighs, buttocks, hips, abdominals, and back.

Our goal is for you to be comfortable walking for 40 to 60 minutes at a 15-minute-mile pace or better. Ideally you'll be motivated to go even faster, cranking it up to 14-, 13-, or even 12-minute miles. That may not sound fast, but keeping up a 12-minutes-per-mile pace is hard work, and going much faster than that is a real challenge. When I'm huffing along at an 11-minute-mile pace, it's almost impossible to believe that an elite race walker's pace is closer to 7 minutes per mile!

SPEED AND TECHNIQUE

To go fast, you need good form, and in this program you'll learn techniques like pumping your arms, pushing off with your toes, and quickening your step to increase your speed.

There's added benefit to walking this way: Research on race walkers suggests that when you get more of your body involved in the motion of walking, the caloric expenditure goes up, even if your speed stays the same. In other words, just by using these techniques you can burn more calories whether or not you walk faster.

This kind of striding requires more concentration and effort than going for a stroll. You're going to have to make a conscious effort to think about what your head, shoulders, arms, and feet are doing. It's okay to yak with your walking partner, but you also need to monitor your pace and form, and push yourself a little.

On the other hand, this is fast walking, not race walking. Don't feel like you have to start waggling your hips and flailing your arms. When you get it right—a quick, natural stride, arms pumping efficiently—it shouldn't look or feel awkward. It's true that the faster you go, the more likely you are to attract a little attention, but believe me, once you get going you don't give a damn what you look like, because you're into it! So stand tall, lift up your head and put some pride in your stride.

A WORD TO THE TORTOISES

Every mother knows that there are some people who simply cannot be rushed, and fast walking won't be everyone's cup of tea. If speeding up is too much of a struggle, or if it makes your muscles sore, you may find your resolve crumbling. You should be able to avoid this by boosting your speed gradually, and allowing your body to adapt to each increase in pace.

If it comes down to a choice between walking slower or not walking at all, by all means slow down! As the Cooper Institute study showed, slower walking is still good for you. If you want to lose weight but you don't want to walk fast, take more frequent, longer walks—an hour or more.

THE PAYOFF

What do you get when you combine consistency and speed?

- *Cardiovascular benefits.* If you're regularly getting your heart rate in your aerobic training zone (which I'll explain in Chapter 3), you're improving your cardiovascular condition. This means lower blood pressure, lower resting heart rate, and increased oxygen delivery to your muscles.
- *Disease prevention.* Several major, long-term studies have found that regular physical activity significantly reduces the risk of *heart disease*. Regular walking can also improve your cholesterol profile. Regular exercise also appears to reduce *hypertension*, and by helping to control your weight, walking can further reduce your risk factors for all of these diseases, as well as *diabetes*. Finally, walking can increase bone mineral content and help prevent *osteoporosis*.
- *Longevity and aging.* Exercise may help you live longer, but even more important is its power to improve the *quality* of life as you age. Recent research suggests that a lot of what we consider aging— weakness, declining aerobic capacity, increased body fat—is really the result of inactivity. It's the "use it or lose it" theory: By staying active, you maintain more lean muscle mass and greater aerobic capacity, thereby staying stronger, longer.

    There are plenty of lifelong walkers in their 70s, 80s, and even 90s who are living evidence for this theory. But studies also show that even completely sedentary 70- and 80-year-olds who start walking programs can significantly improve their aerobic condition.

- *Psychological benefits.* While most health benefits of walking have a long-term payoff, the psychological dividends are paid immediately, in the form of improved mood. By reducing depression, tension, and anxiety, and by increasing feelings of well-being, walking can have a powerful effect on your life.
- *Increased energy.* Although it's difficult to prove in a laboratory, walking seems to make people feel more energetic. Researchers speculate that because walking improves circulation and increases oxygen delivery, while reducing depression and anxiety—known energy sappers—it makes us feel more peppy.
- *Muscle toning.* While we all know there's no such thing as spot reducing, it is a physiological fact that walking, and particularly fast walking, trains and therefore tones the muscles of the legs, particularly the gluteals in your butt and the upper thighs, as well as the abdominals.
- *Calorie burning and weight control.* The evidence about exercise and weight loss is overwhelming. If you want to lose pounds permanently, exercise *must* be part of the program. The reasons are clear: To begin with, you burn calories when you walk. With the fast walking in this program, you're going to maximize that caloric expense. But studies suggest that regular walking also helps with weight loss in other ways. Your metabolism seems to stay slightly higher for a few hours after you stop exercising, burning even more calories. Your appetite, meanwhile, may decrease.

What's more, regular fast walking and a low-fat diet can decrease body fat and increase lean muscle mass. This will increase your resting metabolic rate (RMR), which is the number of calories your body uses for basic maintenance. Compared to fat, muscle tissue is like a calorie furnace: Even when you're not exercising, it burns lots of fuel. (That's why men need more calories then women. With more muscle mass, they burn more fuel every minute.) By walking, you can increase the amount of lean muscle mass in your body and give yourself more ammunition for the fight against weight gain. We'll talk more about weight loss and maintenance in Chapter 5.

GET HOOKED!

More and more, scientists are telling us that our day-to-day habits have a profound effect on the quality and maybe even the length of our lives. There is more evidence than ever that regular physical activity and good eating habits over the course of a lifetime may prevent the diseases that kill many Americans. That's a pretty good reason to give walking a try.

Once you start walking, you'll discover the other reasons, such as what you feel in your body and mind during and after a great walk. It goes something like this:

You start to walk, and as your lungs start to actively move oxygen into and out of your body, the tension you've been holding in your chest all day is exhaled away. You start to concentrate on your walking posture, and you finally manage to relax your shoulders and neck. As you focus on the techniques and sensations of fast walking, the things that were driving you crazy a half-hour earlier slowly slip out of your mind. Soon the rhythm of your steps takes on its own life. Now you're walking hard: You can feel your muscles working, your heart pumping. When you're done, your legs feel light, as though they've been pumped with helium. You feel strong, flexible, and centered.

Now, relaxed and energized, you can get back into your day, feeling good about yourself because you made it happen. You may even find that you sleep better at night when you move your body during the day.

These are the rewards that make it easy to get hooked on walking. And there's no reason to stop, either. Not pregnancy or having children (more on that in Chapter 6); not burn-out or injury, not even aging. With treadmills and mall walking—or just some good foul-weather gear—even bad weather isn't an insurmountable obstacle.

I guess that's what *I* mean when I say that walking is a lifelong activity: With walking, you're set for life.

2

Thinking about Exercise

Before you lace up your walking shoes, I want you to stop for a few minutes and think about your walking program.

I know what you're going to say: "But that's my problem! I *think* about exercise all the time. I just never *do* it." Well, this is a different way to think about exercise. This is applying your mind to a problem: You want to get into the habit of walking regularly. Now how are you going to work it into your life?

In this stage of getting in shape—let's call it "pre-warm-up"—think of your brain as the muscle that needs to do some hard work. If you use your mind before you use your hamstrings, abdominals, and gluteals, you'll get a lot further. Start by creating a workable program for yourself. Later on, you'll have to apply more mental energy to overcome the inevitable obstacles, challenges, and setbacks.

Without your brain, your legs are nowhere. So let's get started on the mental groundwork for this walking program.

CONSISTENCY, *AGAIN*

At the risk of driving you crazy, I'm going to repeat this one more time: Consistency is the key to lifelong fitness, health, and weight control, and the kind of consistency I'm talking about is walking four to six days a week, for a minimum of 30 minutes, and preferably for 40 to 60 minutes. That may sound like a lot right now, but once you get into a routine, I bet you'll find it's manageable. And the rewards for that kind of commitment will be tremendous.

Now you might be thinking, "That Kathy—what a slave driver! I thought three times a week was the recommended amount of aerobic exercise." But according to the American College of Sports Medicine, three times a week is the *minimum* amount required for maintaining cardiovascular fitness. This program is geared for *maximum* results—not only in terms of cardiovascular fitness, but for calorie burning and muscle toning as well. If you're trying to lose weight, three days a week just won't cut it, and the more you walk the better.

One reason walking is so effective is that you *can* do it six days a week. I could never recommend doing step aerobics six days a week, but walking is so forgiving that even if you're out of shape, you can do it every day without worrying about injury. The body is willing to walk regularly. That's why we need to work on the mind.

FROM "HAFTA" TO "WANNA"

It's a lot easier to exercise consistently if you can get from the "hafta" to the "wanna" stage. Right now, you might be thinking, "I *have* to walk four times this week." Ideally you'll get to the point where you think, "I *want* to walk today, because it makes me feel so good." Or, "I *want* to walk today because when I walk I sleep better at night." Half the time, I'm in the "gotta" stage: I've *got* to get away from the house/office/kids and go for a walk!

It's really true that once you start walking regularly, momentum takes over. Because there's so much pleasure, and so little pain, it's incredibly easy to get to the "wanna" stage, if you just give walking a chance to work its magic.

Connie Harris knows what it's like to go from "hafta" to "wanna." I met Connie, a 36-year-old nurse from North Syracuse, New York, when she came to a WALKFIT event in San Francisco. When Connie started WALKFIT, she weighed 237 pounds. "I did very little activity," she told me. "Only what I had to do." At first, walking around the block with her husband was exhausting. Her legs and feet would ache when she was done.

"I really had to force myself out the door, at first," she explained. "But then you start seeing the results. When you're finished, you feel better, not worse, and you start having more energy. And that gets you out the door the next day."

Connie Harris has lost 77 pounds since she started walking, and now she hates to miss a single day. "If something comes up, or if it's raining all day, I really miss it," she says. "I feel like I've cheated myself if I don't walk. Of course, there are still days that I procrastinate, but once I'm out the door, I think, 'Why did I even hesitate?'"

What we're going to do now is chart a course from "hafta" to "wanna." We're going to make a plan to establish a new habit—regular walking. It's like planting a seed: If you put the seed into fertile soil, under the right conditions it will take root and grow. Well, if you start your walking program under the right conditions, it too will take root and grow into a lifelong commitment. I call this "setting yourself up for success."

I think a successful "planting" of new habits requires a four-part strategy:

• Breaking down mental barriers
• Establishing specific, inspirational goals
• Making a plan that you can live with
• Making a commitment to your plan

Let's take them one by one.

BREAKING DOWN BARRIERS

If only changing our habits was as easy as changing our hairstyle. Then we all would have started eating right and exercising a long time ago! The truth is that big changes are always a little scary, whether it's changing jobs or changing habits. It seems that when we were kids, we were a lot more flexible about change.

When I was growing up, my dad was in the military. Every three years our family would pick up and move, usually clear across the country. I'd have to start all over in a new school, making new friends, figuring out which of my clothes were "in" and which ones were totally uncool. Somehow I managed to get through it all, just as most kids adapt to change.

When we get older and have more control over our lives, we tend to try to make life easier by avoiding those big changes. I've had people say to me, "Kathy, if I start exercising, then I have to admit I'm overweight and that I need to change my lifestyle. That just seems too over-whelming for me." When you feel overwhelmed, it's hard to imagine having enough energy to go out and walk every day. It's very important that you start this program feeling motivated and optimistic, not overwhelmed or stressed out.

This is especially true if you have a history of abandoning exercise programs. You may have some bad feelings associated with that. Maybe you feel a little twinge of "I really should . . ." every time you see those athletic shoes buried deep in your closet. When your previous attempts to change petered out, it may have left you with feelings of failure.

Fear of change and failure are often the real factors behind the most common barrier to change: procrastination. "I'll start exercising next week . . . after the holidays . . . when the kids go back to school." We can always find these kinds of situational reasons not to exercise, but I find that the real reasons often lie a little deeper.

That's why it's important to confront these feelings. Until you do, it's hard to get motivated to try again. The thing to remember is this: It may not have worked out before, but this is now. This time *can* be different. This time you're going to set yourself up for success.

Going back to our seedling, think of it this way: Other times, you may have planted your seed in soil that was too rocky (by choosing a kind of exercise that was very hard for you). So then you got a little lax on watering (you didn't like it, so it was hard to stick with it). And so the plant withered.

This time the conditions are going to be very different. By choosing walking, and preparing yourself mentally for this program, you're planting a hardy seedling in good soil. This time, there's no reason that it shouldn't thrive.

ESTABLISHING GOALS

Why do we need to set goals? Because it's hard to get directions when you don't know where you want to go.

I'm about to tell you how to walk, how fast and for how long, but that won't help if you don't know what you want from walking. I want you to start with a good sense of why you're doing this, and where you want to get with it.

I encourage people not only to make goals, but to write them down, and I regularly do this myself. Putting goals on paper makes them more real, and more important. If you make it important, you'll find a way to do it. I also think it helps to make your goals specific. A goal that's too general, such as, "I want to start walking," is easy to overlook, and it's certainly not very motivating.

Put down the book for a moment, and grab a piece of paper and a pen. Start by asking yourself for 10 specific reasons why you want to start a walking program: physical reasons, psychological reasons, spiritual reasons—whatever comes to mind. Write them down, and look at what you've written: Does it inspire you?

Now try ranking your reasons in order of importance. There has to be a balance between the weight of your goal and your reasons for doing it. It takes a big motivation to make a big change. For example, getting rid of some excess flab on your thighs might motivate you for only a few weeks. On the other hand, becoming the kind of person who can successfully change their habits might provide more lasting motivation.

Look at your list again, and ask yourself this: What's going to keep you going when the going gets tough? Work on your reasons until you feel convinced by them.

A word to the wise: If you are trying to lose weight, try to also think of some goals that aren't weight-related, so that your success isn't solely measured in pounds or inches. You *will* lose weight if you walk regularly, but you'll also be getting healthier, and feeling better mentally and physically, even if you lose weight more slowly than you'd hoped. Don't let those triumphs be overshadowed by the number on the scale!

Sometimes it helps to have external goals in addition to the personal reasons you have for starting this program. For example, I get really motivated by speed goals. When I started working on this book, I set myself a walking goal as well: I decided to get my pace down from 12 minutes a mile to 11 minutes a mile. Now that's specific and, believe me, it's very motivating! Each time I go out for a walk, I bring my time down a little, and when I'm done I can hardly wait to come out the next day, because I know I can go faster. Most of us are at least a little competitive, and challenging yourself to increase your walking pace can stoke that competitive fire.

Similarly, you can choose an event as a goal: Perhaps there's a hike that you'd like to do, or a walking vacation. Or maybe there's a 5K or 10K run/walk for charity coming up in your area. With goals like this, you get a great feeling of accomplishment when the event finally arrives. As soon as it's over, you can pick another event or other goal to walk toward.

Whatever reasons you use for starting your program, you *can* get to the point where walking provides its own motivation: When you realize that your body is feeling stronger and your head is clearer, when you discover that you can get away from the stress in your life once a day, when you realize that you're more energetic all day and sleeping better all night, you'll have all the reasons you need.

MAKING A PLAN, AND COMMITTING TO IT

Now that you've done your psychological homework, let's turn to the logistical homework: figuring out when and how walking is going to fit in your life. This includes getting some foreseeable obstacles out of the way ahead of time.

Getting Support

Unfortunately, one major obstacle is people: family, friends, co-workers—anyone who is likely to raise an eyebrow when you take off for an hour to walk. I find that it's best to tell the important people in your life about the commitment you're making, and to make sure they understand how important it is to you. Tell them, "I'm going to be doing this program, and I'm going to need your support and cooperation. This is important for me, but don't worry, I'm not going off the deep end."

People don't have to be a problem, of course. Children make great company on a walk: Put the small ones in a baby backpack or baby jogger, and let the big ones bicycle or roller-skate along. Friends, co-workers, and spouses make great walking partners, too—that is, if they're willing to keep up the pace!

Making Time

When you look at people who exercise consistently, what you notice is that somehow, they always manage to find time, or *make time*, for exercise. It's a question of priorities, of course, but these people know that time is the biggest enemy of fitness: There are never enough hours in the day, and workouts can get squeezed.

That's why you need to decide right now when you are going to walk, and for how long. Make a realistic plan for the coming week, and then commit to those times as if they were appointments with a doctor.

If you're lucky enough to have some flexibility in your schedule, try to exercise at the time of day when you most feel like exercising. My husband, Steve, and I usually feel like exercising at different times of day: for me, it's morning; for Steve, it's midnight. So sometimes we compromise and walk together at four in the afternoon.

Now I may be a morning person, but many people find it easier to exercise in the afternoon. In fact, some interesting studies have found that most people find that it's actually physically easier to exercise in the afternoon. The researchers speculate that daily fluctuations in your body temperature make it easier to get revved up in the afternoon.

If you don't have the luxury of a flexible schedule, you're going to have to be a little more creative. One option is to set the alarm an hour earlier and walk first thing in the morning. (Here's a plus: In the study I just mentioned, the researchers found that the morning workouts felt harder, but they also burned more calories, because your body is a little less efficient in the a.m.). Getting out of bed an hour early still sounds too painful? How about 30 minutes earlier? How about walking during your lunch hour? After dinner? To and from work?

Once you've chosen a time, I want you to stick with it for one week. That's all—just one week. That's how you start to make changes in your life. After a week, you can reassess and adjust your plan.

LIONS AND TIGERS AND BEARS

I talked earlier about setting yourself up for success. In this case, success means sticking with walking for the long haul, making consistent exercise a lifelong habit. If you do the things we just talked about—set *goals* that are important to you, *plan* time for walks, and *commit* to that plan, you're on the right road. But like the Yellow Brick Road in *The Wizard of Oz,* the road to success is not without its perils—along the way, there are "lions and tigers and bears. Oh, my!"

Every now and then, life goes haywire. Maybe the weather gets bad, or your walking partner goes on vacation, or it's February—anything. You don't walk for a whole week, and you're ready to give up; you'll never get back to Kansas. Here's another enthusiasm-killer: The digits on the scale refuse to go down any further or (worse) start moving in the wrong direction.

How do you deal with these challenges when you don't have a lion, a tin man, and a scarecrow cheering you on every step of the way?

Let's take the last challenge first: the scale. This is why I suggest having separate goals for weight loss and walking. If you're walking regularly and sticking to a low-fat diet, you *will* lose weight over time. As you probably already know, weight doesn't always come off in a steady, predictable way. If you're walking fast, you may be replacing fat with lean muscle mass, which could also make your weight loss slower than expected. So you need to be patient, but more importantly, you need to look for positive reinforcement in other places. Instead of relying on the scale, let lower blood pressure, faster walking speed, or the great feeling of lightness in your legs tell you how well you're doing.

When confronted by obstacles, flexibility beats frustration. If your walking partner moves or changes jobs, recruit someone else from the office or neighborhood; you'll be doing a favor for them as well as yourself. When the weather gets bad or the days get short, seek out a gym with a treadmill or an indoor track, or try mall-walking. You can rise to the challenge. You have the power to make it work.

Stay flexible on a daily basis, by keeping a pair of shoes in your bag or in your car. That way, on even those hectic days when your schedule gets wrecked by a traffic jam, a meeting that never happens, or "Sorry, but the doctor is running an hour behind today," you can always score a victory for sanity with a walk.

Getting around those lions and tigers and bears is easier than you think. In fact, I find I get a certain joy from thinking my way out of what seemed to be a hopeless situation, or getting past a trouble spot.

Through it all, keep in mind that your aim is consistency, not perfection. Life is about common sense, about being practical and rational. WALKFIT is as much of a challenge for your brain as it is for your thighs and calves.

REST

Enough about work! Let's talk about rest.

You may find it surprising that I'm going to tell you *not* to exercise, but that's exactly what I'm going to do. Let me explain. Exercise is a stimulus to your body; it's like water to the plant. You water a plant, and between waterings it grows. If you just kept pouring more and more water on it, you wouldn't be doing any good after a while. Eventually you could kill the plant.

Well, your body adapts to walking—by getting stronger and more efficient in its use of oxygen, for example—in between walks. Just as with watering the plant, if you exercise hard every single day you're not doing yourself any good. After a while, you can start to do harm. It's called overtraining.

I learned this the hard way. A few years back, it seemed that I'd turn up in the doctor's office once a year with some sort of sick-as-a-dog symptoms. Usually it was my lungs and chest that were bothering me. Each time, my doctor would ask me what I'd been doing recently. As I painted a picture of the two months leading up to the visit, it usually involved training for a video and consistently working out hard. Whenever I felt tired, I'd exercise, thinking it would energize me. What I was really doing was overtraining, and making myself sick in the process. I'd end up with some sort of lung infection and be flat on my back for a week. It would be a month before I could get back to full strength.

Ordinarily overtraining isn't a big concern for walkers. Walking is a forgiving activity that doesn't usually cause overuse injuries. But at a fast WALKFIT pace, it is possible to overdo it. The harder you walk relative to your current level of fitness, the more important it is to allow your body time to adapt and recover.

You have to listen to your body and know when it's time to take a rest. Exercise should pick up your energy level: Once you're in shape, it's a bad sign to feel excessively tired after a walk. Persistent tiredness, heaviness in your legs, irritability, sleeplessness, and minor injuries that don't heal are all signs of too much exercise. Another way to tell if you've overdone it is to take your heart rate first thing in the morning. Usually, it stays about the same day in and day out. A sudden rise in your resting heart rate may mean you're pushing too hard.

These kinds of symptoms would probably occur only if you were walking at a very fast pace five days a week. The easiest way to avoid any problems is to limit your hard workouts to two to three times per week. On the other days, reduce either your speed or your distance. If you're walking a lot and your legs start to feel a little heavy, or if you feel sluggish, take a day off. If your pace gets fast enough—13-minute miles or better—it's a good idea to plan at least two easy days and one day off per week.

I learned the hard way. You can incorporate rest right from the beginning to keep yourself healthy.

There's another kind of overdoing it that's even more common: burn-out. I find it's less of a problem with walking than with other activities, but there may be times when the idea of a spin around the usual route leaves you flatter than warm ginger ale.

When I'm feeling uninspired, I can sometimes psych myself up by telling myself I'm *not* going out for 4 miles today. I tell myself I'm just going for a walk, and I give myself an out: If after 10 minutes I'm zonked and I can't get into it, I can give up. I go out the door thinking I have to walk for only 10 minutes, but I usually end up feeling great and doing the entire walk.

A less devious option is just to break the monotony by doing something different: Change your route, or call a friend and suggest taking a walk. Go for a moonlight walk. Or try a little cross-training: Go for a swim or a bike ride. Pop in an exercise video. In Chapter 7, you'll find suggestions for adding variety and challenge to your walking routine.

Remember, flexibility beats frustration, and it beats burn-out, too. On those days when your motivation is a quart low, it's a real triumph to get out and do something!

WHEN THE MIND LEADS, THE BODY FOLLOWS

I called this chapter "Thinking about Exercise" because while walking is a physical activity, changing your habits is a mental process. Your body doesn't get stronger and fitter without a lot of help from your mind. Spend some mental energy planning your walking program. Then be prepared to use your head to creatively handle the challenges that inevitably arise as you try to change your habits.

3

The WALKFIT
Program

WALKFIT is a two-phase program in which the first phase, Foundation, gets you prepared for the fast walking in phase two, Workout. In both phases, you'll learn new techniques for boosting your walking speed. As you master these techniques, and your fitness increases, you'll be able to walk faster and farther.

Foundation. This is where you lay the groundwork for fast, effective walking. Learning the Foundation basics of posture, breathing, relaxation, and foot action will make it easier to increase your pace later on. Foundation is also where you build your fitness base, by gradually boosting the frequency, length, and speed of your walks. When you're more fit, Foundation techniques are used for warm-up and cool-down.

Workout. Here you'll build on your Foundation with techniques that boost not only your speed but your calorie burn and muscle toning as well. Workout techniques help you comfortably move up to the 15-minute-mile WALKFIT pace. As your fitness increases, you'll spend more and more of your walking time in Workout.

As you get more comfortable with fast walking, you may want to challenge yourself a little more, and crank up your pace. Using Foundation techniques, you can increase your pace to 12-minute miles or faster—taking walking to its limits in terms of aerobic conditioning, muscle toning, and calorie burning. You'll learn to handle this high-intensity walking with interval training, which I'll explain later on.

GUIDING YOUR WALKS

For safe and efficient walks, it's important to know how hard you're working. That means monitoring your "exercise intensity." If it's too low, you're shortchanging yourself, because you could be getting a lot more out of your time spent walking. On the other hand, if it's too high you're making things difficult for yourself, and you'll tire out too quickly.

There are three ways to monitor exercise intensity: 1) target heart rate (THR); 2) rate of perceived exertion (RPE); and 3) the "talk test."

Target Heart Rate

You may be familiar with THR, which is actually a range of heart rates, determined by your age, within which you get an effective aerobic workout. For normal, healthy people, the aerobic training zone is between 60 percent and 80 percent of maximum heart rate. (See the chart on p. 33.)

Your maximum heart rate is calculated by subtracting your age from 220.

Target Training Zones

Age	Target Zone
20	120–160
25	117–156
30	114–152
35	111–148
40	108–144
45	105–140
50	102–136
55	99–132
60	96–128
65	93–124
70	90–120
75 +	87–116

So if you're 40, your maximum heart rate is 180, give or take a few beats. To calculate your target heart rate for aerobic training, you take 60 percent of 180 (which is 108) for the low end, and 80 percent of 180 (which is 144) for the high end. Then you try to walk at a pace that keeps your heart rate above 108, but below 144.

Why? Because a heart rate of less than 60 percent of your maximum means the exercise probably isn't challenging enough to increase your aerobic fitness. A heart rate above 80 percent of maximum is good for certain kinds of training, but it's not optimal for the kind of sustained calorie burn and cardiovascular conditioning we're after.

To use THR as a guide, find your training zone on the chart, and check your heart rate periodically during your walks. Your first check should be after your warm-up: about 10 minutes into your walk. Measure your heart rate by taking your pulse at your neck or wrist. Count heart-beats for 10 seconds (starting with zero), then multiply that by 6. If your heart rate is below your target zone, you need to speed up and/or increase your arm swing. If your heart rate is above the zone, slow down. Recheck a few minutes after adjusting your pace. You can measure THR again in the middle and at the end of your walk.

If you're just getting into shape, keep your heart rate closer to 60 percent of your maximum. When you start feeling more comfortable with exercise, you can gradually increase the intensity. If you add interval training to your workouts (see below), your pulse may climb above 80 percent.

Heart-rate monitors are a convenient way to track your pulse. These devices usually consist of a chest strap, which measures your heart rate, and a monitor, which displays the figure. You get constant, instant feedback from them so you don't have to stop and take a pulse. But they're also expensive ($125 and up), and unnecessary for general fitness training.

Rate of Perceived Exertion

RPE is a way to estimate how hard you're working by simply taking stock of how you're feeling—changes in breathing, heart rate, sweating, and fatigue—and then rating those sensations on a scale from 6 ("very, very light") to 20 ("very, very hard"). The advantage of RPE over pulse taking is that you don't have to stop exercising to measure it.

To rate your perceived exertion, just think about how you feel as you're walking: Do your legs feel like they're hardly working, or do they hurt? Are you breathing hard?

Is your heart pounding? Are you sweating? Then assign a number to your observation, as follows:

6–8	Very, very light exertion	13–14 Somewhat hard
9–10	Very light	15–16 Hard
11–12	Moderate	17–18 Very hard
		19–20 Very, very hard

During your walks, try to stay in the 13 to 16 range. (Beginning exercisers should be closer to 13.) Warm-up and cool-down should be between 10 and 12. The key to using RPE is to practice with it, because you're comparing how you feel on any given day to how you've felt on other days. The more experience you have with aerobic exercise, the easier it is to understand and use RPE.

The Talk Test

This is the easiest and least technical way to monitor intensity. You should be walking hard enough so that you can talk but find it a little bit difficult to carry on a conversation—you may need to take deep breaths between sentences, for example. If you're so out of breath that you can't complete a sentence, slow down. If you're chatting as easily as if you were sitting on the couch, get moving!

Finally, if at any point you feel undue pain, fatigue, or shortness of breath, slow down. If you feel nausea or dizziness, stop immediately.

FOUNDATION

In Foundation, we're going to focus on body position, breathing, and foot action. But let's start with some whole-body, general ideas about relaxation and exercise.

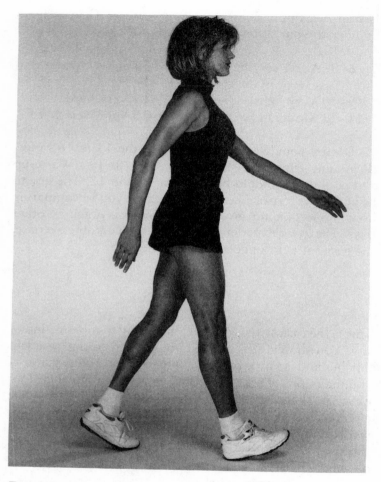

Foundation begins with good walking posture. Your head is erect, with eyes focused forward, your shoulders are down and back, and your abdominals are contracted. Notice that the stride length is comfortable—not exaggerated. Your arms are swinging freely, and the left arm is moving forward with the right leg. As your right heel strikes the ground, the toes of your left foot are beginning to push off.

Imagine walking with an egg in your hand: If you don't grip it, you'll drop it. If you grip it too hard, you'll smash it. Exercise calls for that kind of balance. The trick is to be relaxed, so you don't get fatigued by unnecessary muscle tension, but without being limp as a wet noodle. For comfortable, efficient exercise, strive for controlled, fluid motions—not stiffness.

Let's use your arms as an example: If there's tension in your arm, shoulder and neck muscles, you'll get tired and achy. On the other hand, if your arms are flailing or flopping at your sides, you're wasting energy that should be propelling you forward. The proper balance is an efficient, compact arm swing, without excess tension in the shoulders.

FOUNDATION TECHNIQUES

POSTURE

Keep in mind our goal of being relaxed but ready to go. Now, stand tall. Imagine a string coming out of the top of your head, pulling you up. Then tilt that long body forward *slightly*, tilting from the ankles, not the hips or the waist. Contract your abdominals so that your pelvis shifts forward slightly, to keep your spine in a neutral position. Don't arch your lower back or stick your butt out.

HEAD POSITION

Your head should be erect, not cocked or tilted to one side. Lift your chin and chest and focus your eyes ahead of you—not at your feet—to take unnecessary strain off your neck.

SHOULDERS

Your shoulders should be down and back, opening up your chest for easier, deeper breathing. It's a natural position— there's no need to pull your shoulders back like chicken wings. As you walk, check your shoulders regularly: Are you starting to slouch? Are your shoulders creeping up toward your ears? If they are, a few shrugs or shoulder rolls will get 'em back down.

ARMS

Let your arms swing freely, but with purpose: It improves balance, increases circulation, and burns more calories. Your arms move in opposition to your legs: The right leg and left arm always move together. Swing your arms forward, not across your body. Imagine your body (viewed from the side) on a clock face, with your head at 12 o'clock: Your arms should swing from about 7 o'clock (just behind your hips) to 4 o'clock (about belly-button height).

FEET

Strike the ground with your heel, and let your foot roll forward naturally. At the end of the stride, instead of just letting your foot leave the ground, really push off with your toes, to actively propel your body forward. Use the stride length that's comfortable for you—your normal walking stride. *Don't overstride.* Taking unnaturally long strides will wear you out quickly.

Mind Your Form, with RACES

Throughout your walks, periodically check your body position. Make a habit of good technique, by memorizing this Foundation checklist. I've made up a memory cue to help you remember these important techniques: RACES.

Roll those feet from heel to toe
Arms swing with purpose
Contract your abdominals
Eyes straight ahead
Shoulders down and back

WORKOUT

Now we're going to add on to the Foundation you've established—good walking posture, tight abdominals, deep breathing, heel strike, and toe push-off—with techniques for increasing your speed. In Workout, you can start to pick up the pace: 13 to 15 minutes per mile is an excellent fitness walking pace, and you can go faster than that, if you want to. Keep in mind, though, that you'll burn more calories using these techniques even if you don't walk a whole lot faster.

WORKOUT TECHNIQUES

ARM SWING

Since your arms and legs work in unison, your legs can't speed up unless your arms do. To get your arms pumping more quickly, start by putting a 90-degree bend in your elbow and holding your hands in a loose fist. Now, for the pump:

- Swing forward, not side to side, keeping your elbows close to your sides. Your hands will end up in front of your body, but don't let your right hand cross over to the left side of your body, or vice versa.
- On the backswing, your hand should reach your hipbone, but it shouldn't go behind you. Coming forward, your hand shouldn't go above chest height.
- For a controlled, efficient pumping action, visualize the shafts that drive the wheels of a locomotive. They move forward and back, forward and back, in an almost circular motion, and that's what your arms should be doing.

FEET

Use the same rolling, heel-toe motion as in Foundation. Concentrate on pushing off with your toes to increase your pace, and *actively pull up your toes* as your leg swings forward. At faster paces, if you don't pull up the toes, you'll start catching them on the ground.

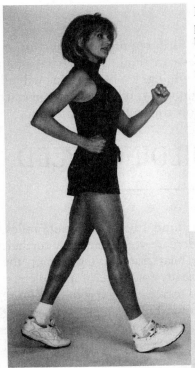

In Workout, maintain that good posture, and add a 90-degree bend in the elbow, holding your hands in a loose fist. On the backswing, notice that your right hand goes only as far as your hipbone—it doesn't go behind the body. The left hand, which is swinging forward, reaches chest height. Notice the angle in the right foot as the heel strikes the ground. You've really got to pull up on those toes!

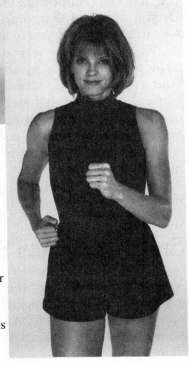

Looking at the arm action from the front, you see that your arms swing in front of your body, but not across it. Imagine a line stretching from your nose to your belly button: Your hands should reach chest height right on that line. Notice also that your elbows stay close to your sides as your arms pump forward and back.

CONCENTRATION

Maintaining good Workout form requires a lot of concentration. You're going to have to think about what your arms, legs, hips, and feet are doing. Eventually this will all become habit, but in the beginning you'll find that you start slowing down when you stop concentrating on form.

TIPS FOR BUILDING SPEED

At a certain point, usually around 13- or 14-minute miles, you may find it difficult to increase your speed any further. Or you may find that your heart rate isn't going up the way it used to, and you're ready for more of a challenge.

We know that the way to increase speed is to take more steps per minute, *not* by taking bigger steps. But moving your legs that quickly takes an enormous amount of effort: In fact, at 5 MPH, it's much more efficient to run—and cover more ground with each stride—than it is to walk. So you actually use more energy, and burn more calories, walking a 12-minute mile than running a 12-minute mile.

When you're ready to crank it up to 12 minutes per mile, here's how to get your body to move that fast:

SPEED UP THE ARM SWING

You can really add to your forward momentum—and get some significant upper-body exercise—by pumping your arms more quickly. As you start to go a little faster, your arms will swing across your body slightly, and that's okay.

WALK THE LINE

Up until now, you've been walking with your feet parallel. To increase your speed, try to make your feet land one in front of the other, so you're walking a straight line. If you were walking on an actual line, just the inside of your foot (the instep) would touch the line: Your feet shouldn't cross over. Check yourself by walking an actual line: a painted lane line on a track or a crack in the pavement, for example.

"Walking the line" forces you to rotate your pelvis and extend your hips slightly, which lengthens your stride a little. At faster speeds, you'll get some front-to-back rotation in your pelvis. Don't consciously try to waggle your hips or exaggerate the motion: Just align your footsteps, leading with your heels, and stay loose in your pelvis as your hips follow where your legs lead.

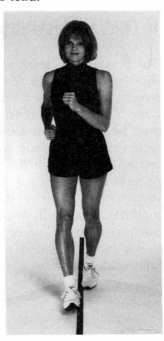

At the interval pace, you're walking the line, with your feet landing directly in front of one another. The line on the floor shows that only the inside edge of the foot reaches the line. Also notice that the left arm is now crossing over *slightly* to the right side of the body. Maintain good posture as your speed increases— keep your head up, and your shoulders down and back.

A note to men: Since you have less hip swivel in your normal walking gait than women do, this technique can be more difficult for you. Make a conscious effort to stay loose in your hips and to let your pelvis rotate. The leg and hip stretches in Chapter 8 will also help increase your range of motion.

Squeeze Your Glutes

Your gluteals are the muscles in your butt, just above your hamstrings. At the end of each stride, as you're pushing off with your toes, squeeze the gluteals in the same leg. This helps draw the leg back, which increases your speed and conditions the muscles in the butt.

Interval Training

The best way to learn to walk this fast is to practice for short stretches, with rest periods at a slower pace in between. This is called "interval training." By alternating intervals of high-intensity effort with recovery periods, your heart, lungs, and muscles can work harder for short spurts than they could work continuously. Start with 30-second intervals of high-intensity walking, with 30 seconds of recovery in between. These high-intensity intervals can dramatically improve your fitness, but they're very demanding. Eventually you'll be able to maintain that high-intensity pace for longer and longer periods of time. You'll find a sample interval workout in the Level V program, later in the chapter.

WALKFIT PROGRAMS

Now that you've got the techniques, what are you going to do with them? People who prefer less-structured exercise can simply go out and walk: Just keep in mind the goal of walking 40 to 60 minutes, and, using THR, RPE, or the talk test as your guide, try to keep up your intensity. You should end up walking somewhere between 2.0 and 4.5 miles.

If you prefer a little more structure, I've created five WALKFIT workouts for different levels of fitness. If you are inactive or have any pre-existing medical conditions, you should check with your doctor before starting in Level I. If you're reasonably active and in good health, with no pre-existing cardiovascular or musculo-skeletal conditions, it's still a good idea to check with your doctor, and you can probably start with Level II or III. If you're a regular exerciser (30 to 40 minutes of aerobic activity at least four times a week), you can start with Level IV.

Each WALKFIT level has a fitness goal, measured in minutes per mile. When you meet that goal, you're ready to move on to the next level. In general, it should take 6 to 12 weeks to meet these goals, but don't be discouraged if it takes longer.

If you're following these programs, it's important and helpful to know distances and paces. If you're not walking on a track, drive your walking route in your car and figure out where the mile markers are. If you can't drive your route, because it's in a park, for example, figure it out with a map.

As you're walking, check your time at the mile markers. If you're off your pace, pick it up. Using mile markers and a watch is a big help when you're walking and talking. It's easy to forget about your pace when you're yakking, as I know from walking with my husband, Steve. We have mile markers around our neighborhood, and they keep us honest.

FITNESS SELF-TEST

You can also find out which program is best for you by testing your fitness level with the 1-mile walk test. This self-test will get you started in the right place, and it will also give you a baseline against which you can see yourself improve over the coming weeks and months. Watching your time improve is a great motivator.

What You Need: A track or a flat mile course that you've measured in your neighborhood, and a watch with a stopwatch capacity. You'll also need to know your target heart rate.

What To Do: Warm up for at least eight minutes, then start your timer and walk 1 mile at a brisk pace. Try to keep up a pace that makes you breathe a little bit hard—not huffing and puffing, though. When you finish the mile, record the time and check your heart rate: Were you in your training zone? If so, your mile time is a valid starting point.

- If your heart rate was below your training zone and you didn't feel exhausted by your effort, try the walk again after a day of rest, and pick up the pace.
- If your heart rate was above your training zone, you're pushing too hard. Try the self-test again after a day of rest, but stop halfway through to check your heart rate. If you're above your zone, slow down. At the end of your walk, subtract the amount of time it took to take your pulse from your total walking time.

LEVELS I–V

Level I. If your test-mile time was over 24 minutes (or if you cannot walk 1 mile):

- Start in Foundation, walking as long as you can, up to 30 or 40 minutes, including warm-up and cool-down.
- After warming up at a comfortable pace for about 10 minutes, try to increase your pace slightly, so that you're walking faster than your around-town pace. For the last 10 minutes of your walk, cool down by gradually slowing your pace.
- Monitor your intensity using one of the methods above. Stay closer to 60 percent of your maximum heart rate, or keep your RPE down around 13.
- Walk four to six times per week, or as often as you can. Walk as far as you can, eventually working up to 1.25 to 1.75 miles.
- Your goal is to walk 1.5 miles in less than 36 minutes.

Level II. If your test-mile time was 20:00 to 23:59 minutes:

- Start in Foundation, walking for at least 30 minutes, preferably 40 or 60. Total time includes warm-up and cool-down.
- After a 10-minute warm-up, try to increase your pace slightly and hold that pace for the remainder of your walk. Make a conscious effort to walk at a pace that's faster than your walk-around-town pace. Cool down for 10 minutes by gradually slowing your pace.
- Monitor your intensity using one of the methods above. Aim for 60 to 70 percent of your maximum heart rate, or an RPE of about 15.
- Walk four to six times per week, covering 1.5 to 3 miles.
- Your goal is to walk 2 miles in less than 40 minutes.

Level III. If your test-mile time was 16:00 to 19:59 minutes:

- Start with two weeks in Foundation. Walk for 40 to 60 minutes, including warm-up and cool-down.
- After two weeks, walk for 10 minutes in Foundation, then move into Workout for 20 to 30 minutes. Cool down for 10 minutes by gradually slowing from Workout back to Foundation. A typical workout would look like this:

> 10 minutes: Foundation warm-up
> 10–15 minutes: Workout, at a moderate pace
> 10–15 minutes: Increase to a faster Workout pace
> 10 minutes: Cool-down from Workout to Foundation

- Monitor your intensity using one of the methods above. Aim for 60 to 75 percent of your maximum heart rate, or an RPE of 14 to 16.
- Walk four to six times per week, covering 2 to 3.75 miles.
- Your goal is to walk 3 miles in less than 48 minutes.

Level IV. If your test-mile time was 13:00 to 15:59 minutes:

- Start with a 10-minute warm-up in Foundation. Then go into Workout for 30 to 40 minutes, gradually increasing your pace. Cool down for 10 minutes by slowing from Workout back to Foundation. A typical workout would look like this:

  10 minutes: Foundation warm-up
  15 minutes: Workout, at a moderate pace
  15 minutes: Increase to a faster Workout pace
  10 minutes: Cool-down from Workout to
  Foundation pace

- Monitor your intensity using one of the methods above. Aim for 60 percent to 80 percent of your maximum heart rate, or an RPE of 14 to 16. Walking at 80 percent or an RPE of 16 every day is an invitation to burn-out: Include a couple of lower-intensity walks each week.
- Walk four to six times per week, covering 3 to 4.5 miles.
- Your goal is to walk 3 miles in 39 minutes.

Level V. If your test-mile time was under 12:59 minutes:

• Start in Foundation for an 8-minute warm-up. Go into Workout for 20 minutes. Follow with intervals: 45 seconds of hard walking—as fast as you can— alternating with 45 seconds in easy Workout. Start with 6 minutes of intervals (that's four sets: four hard ones, four easy ones), followed by 6 minutes of steady, fast walking, and another 6 minutes of intervals. It looks like this:

> 8 minutes: Foundation warm-up
> 20 minutes: Workout
> 6 minutes: 8 × 45-second fast/easy intervals
> 6 minutes: Workout
> 6 minutes: 8 × 45-second fast/easy intervals

Cool down for 10 minutes by gradually slowing from Workout back to Foundation. Don't do intervals more than three times per week. On the other days, substitute 18 more minutes in Workout for the interval period.

As you become more fit, you can increase either the length of your intervals (keeping a one-to-one ratio between hard and easy) or the number of intervals you do. For example, you could do sets of six 1-minute intervals (1 minute hard, 1 minute easy). Or do 9 minutes worth of 45-second intervals.

• Monitor your intensity using one of the methods above. Aim for 60 percent to 85 percent (during intervals) of your maximum heart rate, or an RPE of 14 to 16 (18 during intervals). Include at least two easy days per week, where your THR stays at 70 or below, or your RPE stays below 15.

• Walk four to six times per week, from 3 to 5 miles.
• Your goal is to be able to hold a 12-minute-mile pace for 3 to 5 miles.

WARM-UP AND COOL-DOWN TIPS

Whether or not you follow one of these programs, all of your walks should include warm-up and cool-down periods.

The best way to warm up is simply to start at an easy Foundation pace and gradually increase your speed. This lets your muscles and joints get ready for the demands of fast walking, and it allows your heart rate and circulation to increase slowly and safely. A warm-up is also a chance to focus your mind on what you're doing and let other concerns slip away. Use warm-up time to check in with your body: How do those feet feel? How are the shins and the shoulders? Does anything feel unusually tight today?

Warm-up time varies from individual to individual and even from day to day. Some days I get loose in no time, while other days it takes me longer. Generally, 8 to 12 minutes should do the trick.

A cool-down at the end of your walk allows your heart and circulation to slowly return to normal. When you stop exercising, the amount of oxygen you're inhaling drops sharply. This can sometimes catch your body by surprise, and the result is dizziness. A cool-down lets your body slowly adjust to the lowered oxygen intake.

There's a natural tendency to forget about form during your cool-down, to relax (Yippee! I'm done!) and immediately slouch. Try to maintain good form and posture all the way through. In fact, why not maintain that good posture all day long?

About Shin Pain

A lot of people experience some pain in their shins when they start walking fast. This is a result of pulling up on your toes (also known as dorsi-flexion). If you've ever had shin splints—a painful, chronic injury—you may worry when your shins start to hurt. But the discomfort you feel when you start walking fast is entirely different, and it's normal: You're using muscles that don't usually work very hard, and they're getting a little sore. Don't get scared away by the initial discomfort. Your muscles will adapt to the demands within two to three weeks, as long as you don't do too much, too soon.

Some people find that their shins bother them early in the walk, but then the discomfort goes away when they warm up. You may want to stop and stretch your shins (see the shin stretches in Chapter 8) after you've warmed up. Stretch your shins thoroughly after cooldown as well.

If the problem persists, you may be pulling up your toes too much. You need to pull them up so they clear the ground as your leg swings under your body, but you don't have to exaggerate it.

If you continue to be bothered by pain, especially if your shins hurt *after* your walk, don't push it. Consider a visit to your doctor. If it doesn't hurt to walk at a slower pace, ease off for a few days, and then try increasing your speed very gradually. Use interval training to allow your shins to gradually adapt to higher demands.

You can also ice your shins after walking to relieve the discomfort and promote healing. I learned this trick from Maryanne Torrellas, a six-time national champion race walker. Maryanne, who can walk a mile in an incredible 6 minutes, 30 seconds, suggests using an ice massage on your shins:

Use ice cubes, or freeze water in a paper cup and then tear off the paper. Move the ice briskly over the surface of your shin. "You don't want to just leave the ice sitting on one spot, because you don't have much skin protecting that muscle," says Torrellas. Ice for five minutes, then stop for five minutes, then ice for five minutes more.

Torrellas also recommends massaging your shins: "Use your thumb to press along the muscle, starting from the bottom of your ankle and going all the way up to just below your knee."

Finally, she offers this strengthening exercise for your shins. You can do this a few times a week, after you've warmed up your shins with a few minutes of walking:

Sit with your legs extended in front of you and your toes pointing up. Hold the ends of a towel in your hands, and place the towel on the ball of your foot. Slowly extend your foot until your toes are pointed, providing *light* resistance with the towel. Don't overload the muscle—make it about a 50 percent effort. Do three sets of 10, working one leg at a time.

STRETCHING

There's no doubt in my mind that stretching helps your body exercise more comfortably. In Chapter 8, I've created a stretching program designed specifically to complement the WALKFIT program. Take time to learn the stretches and make them a regular part of your WALKFIT workouts.

4

≡

Tricks of the Trade:
Walking in Comfort
and Safety

You've probably suspected that exercise is just plain easier for some people than it is for others. Well, it's true, but the reasons aren't only great genes and abnormal energy levels. People who work out regularly know certain tricks for making their bodies feel good. They take care of the little things, like drinking plenty of water, having good shoes and socks, and wearing clothing that's comfortable and appropriate for the weather. I want to share some of the secrets of safe, comfortable exercise with you. You'll find these tricks of the trade can take you a long way.

WALKING SHOES

It is certainly not news to you that good athletic shoes cost a small fortune these days. You may have grown up in eight-dollar Keds, but today the price of comfort and performance runs from about $50 to $80. Generally you get what you pay for. Shoes that cost less than $40 usually have a host of vices: Either they fall apart quickly, or they're not well cushioned or they don't provide enough support.

While walking isn't high-impact, like running or aerobics, you still want a supportive, shock-absorbing shoe. In a 3-mile walk at a 4-MPH pace, your feet will hit the ground roughly 7,500 times. Without good shock absorption, your feet are going to feel a bit beat up after that many ground strikes. You'll walk a lot of miles in this program: Make those miles more comfortable by putting your feet in good shoes.

Fit should be your first priority: The shoe should hug your heel, and the shoe's arch support should hit your instep in the right place. The front of the shoe should be roomy enough that you can wiggle your toes and your big toe doesn't bump into the front of the shoe. Several manufacturers make wide and narrow sizes for hard-to-fit feet.

After fit, what should you look for?

- High-quality midsoles (the shock-absorbing part of the sole), made of materials like polyurethane, or special inserts like gel or air, will hold up better under heavy mileage. Less-expensive shoes may feel good and cushy when you first put them on, but after a few weeks of walking in them, the shock absorption will decline rapidly. With heavy use, the midsoles will flatten out in a month or two, leaving precious little between you and the pavement.
- A durable outsole (the tread that contacts the pavement) made of carbon rubber will offer better traction and won't wear out as quickly.

A good walking shoe will also make it easier to master the techniques that we covered in Chapter 3. Here's why:

• *Toe push-off:* A good walking shoe has a flexible forefoot (the part of the shoe underneath the ball of your foot), which makes it easier to flex your foot and push off at the end of your stride.

   A wide toe-box (the front part of the shoe, where your toes sit) also helps, because when your weight rolls onto your toes, they spread out. If there isn't ample room in the toe-box, your feet will feel pinched.

• *Heel strike:* Since you're leading with and landing on your heel, a stable, well-cushioned heel will absorb the impact and help keep your feet rolling smoothly forward.

• *Heel-to-toe-roll:* Some shoes have features like a beveled heel, or a "rocker" shape, designed to help your foot along in the heel-to-toe rolling motion of a good walking stride.

A good shoe can also help correct imbalances in your own stride. Many people's feet either pronate (roll in) or supinate (roll out) when they walk. To see if you have either of these tendencies, look at the bottom of an old pair of shoes: Does the tread wear evenly? If not, is it more worn down on the inside of your foot, near the arch, or on the outside? If the inside is worn, you tend to pronate. If the outside wears faster, you tend to supinate.

   If you're walking a lot of miles, pronation and supination can (but don't always) cause pain in your feet or legs. Some shoes are designed to correct these tendencies with strategic placement of support. If you suspect that you pronate or supinate excessively, your best bet is to go to a running specialty store (they all carry walking shoes) and get advice from an experienced salesperson. Or check out the walking shoe buyer's guides in magazines: These are useful to any shoe shopper, and they identify good shoes for correcting foot problems.

ORTHOTICS

If your feet hurt a lot when you walk, you may have a structural problem, like flat feet or high arches. If a certain part of your foot isn't supporting you the way it's supposed to, other parts of your foot and leg end up working harder. This can result in cramping, pain, or injury anywhere from the ball of your foot to your heel. Good shoes can correct these problems to an extent, but some people need orthotics—either over-the-counter or prescription footbeds that compensate for the weaknesses in your feet. Walking shouldn't cause foot pain. If it does, see a doctor or podiatrist about corrective orthotics, so you can walk in complete comfort.

SOCKS

I've seen people spend $70 on a great pair of walking shoes, and then wear cheap, thin cotton socks and wonder why they get blisters. Cotton socks hold dampness, which makes them rub, causing blisters and "hot spots." If your feet sweat a lot, or if you have problems with blisters, you'll be much more comfortable in socks made of polyester or a polyester blend. There are lots of poly/cotton- or poly/wool-blend athletic socks out there with great features like extra padding around the heel and toe, and "wicking" fibers that move moisture away from your skin.

HYDRATION

Water is the body's most important fuel: It's crucial to your safety in hot, humid weather, it helps keep your energy up, and it can stave off muscle cramps.

When you don't take in enough water, your blood volume actually decreases, which means your circulatory system carries less oxygen and fewer nutrients to your organs, and removes less carbon dioxide. As a result, it's harder to exercise: Your body starts to drag, and you may overheat.

When you work out, you can lose up to two quarts of water per hour through sweat and exhaled moisture. It's easy to get dehydrated, especially if you're not well hydrated to begin with. On hot, humid days, the problem can get out of hand, and turn into a case of heat exhaustion or heat stroke.

Dizziness, nausea, confusion, headache, goose bumps, and muscle cramping are all indications of the early stages of heat stroke. If you experience any of these warning signs, stop exercising, get out of the sun, and drink some water immediately.

People over age 50 should be especially cautious in the hot weather, because your body becomes less heat-tolerant as you age. You're also at a greater risk for heat stroke if you are very overweight, have heart disease, or have ever had heat stroke before. Finally, certain medications can affect your heat tolerance; check with your doctor or pharmacist before exercising in hot, humid weather.

Make a habit of drinking a pint of water in the 30 minutes before you start to walk, regardless of the weather. When it's hot, also try to drink about 4 ounces (a few sips) every 15 minutes during your walking, even if you're not thirsty. If there's no water fountain on your route, take a water bottle with you in a fanny pack or a waist-belt water-bottle carrier. Wearing loose-fitting, light-colored clothing and seeking shady routes will also help prevent heat stroke.

People often ask me if there's any difference between water and fluid replacement drinks like Gatorade. According to the exercise scientists, water is simplest and best, unless you're going to be exercising at a high intensity for more than 90 minutes. For very long outings, you may need some additional salt, potassium, and carbohydrate as well as water. Unless you're planning a long hike, you'll be all set with H_2O.

MUSCLE CRAMPS

Muscle cramps don't strike only in the heat. Doctors aren't really sure why some people are more susceptible to cramps than others, but they do have some clues.

• Dehydration usually plays a role in cramping. If you get cramps in your calves or feet (the most common sites for exercise-related cramps) while exercising or afterward, try drinking more water.
• Some cramps are related to mineral imbalances, so a balanced diet and/or a multimineral supplement may help. A low-calorie diet, particularly if it's not well-balanced nutritionally, combined with exercise is a recipe for cramps: Dieters should make an extra effort to drink plenty of water and may also consider multivitamins and minerals.
• Change seems to trigger cramps, whether it's a change in your level of activity, a change in shoes, or a change in training—if you start doing intervals or walking hills, for example. Again, drinking water may help, along with gentle muscle stretching before and after exercise.

If you do get a calf cramp, you can release it by pulling up on your toes, which forces the muscle to relax. Massaging the muscle and applying ice will also help to relieve the cramping.

EXERCISE AND POLLUTION

Exercising in polluted air is simply not good for you. When you walk, your breathing rate increases, so if there's something bad in the air, you're breathing more of it.

One of the worst things in the air is ozone (which is completely unrelated to the ozone layer you hear so much about). Ozone is formed when car exhaust reacts with sunlight, and it can float through the air a long way from its source, i.e., cars. According to statistics from the Environmental Protection Agency, ozone levels are unacceptable not just in big cities like Los Angeles and New York, but in highly populated areas in nearly every state in the country.

Ozone pollution is worst on sunny days at midday and immediately after rush hour, and the air is usually best early in the morning. Chest pain, coughing, and wheezing are signs of ozone-related irritation. If you live in even a small city, and you experience these symptoms when exercising on a sunny day, take the hint and schedule your walks for earlier or later in the day.

There are other pollutants besides ozone that should be avoided. In general, keeping some distance—a few hundred yards—between yourself and heavily trafficked roads is a good idea. It's a lot more peaceful as well.

COLD WEATHER

If it's not one thing, it's another: If you're not worried about heat stroke and ozone pollution, you probably have to contend with wind chill, icy sidewalks, and snow banks. But just because it's cold doesn't mean you have to hibernate for the winter. You can walk indoors on a treadmill, of course, but a walk in the crisp winter air can be a real treat, as long as you're well prepared.

The key is to dress the part, and that means layering. The most common mistake people make when exercising in the cold is *over*dressing. They put on too much clothing, and when they start walking, they overheat. Then they start to sweat, and wet skin is a real liability in the cold air. Dampness increases the rate of heat loss, and if that warm moisture on your body turns cold, you're at risk for hypothermia. Shivering and feeling sluggish are warning signs of hypothermia.

If you layer properly, you won't overheat because you can just open zippers or shed clothes as you warm up. Usually you'll want two or three layers on your upper body, and just one layer (two if it's really chilly) on your legs. It's okay to be a little on the cool side for the first 10 minutes of your walk. That way, as soon as your body starts generating some heat, you'll be perfectly comfortable.

- *Bottom layer:* A thin layer, like exercise tights or long underwear made of a quick-drying fabric like polypropylene. Avoid cotton, which absorbs sweat and keeps it near your body.
- *Middle layer:* Insulation, like a sweater or polar (polyester) fleece. A neck zipper is helpful on this layer, so you can open it up a little if you start to overheat.
- *Top layer:* A water-resistant, wind-resistant jacket or anorak, with a zipper so you can do some climate control. Start out zipped up, then unzip to let excess heat escape. Your outer layer should have a hood for wind and rain protection.
- Hands and feet are likely trouble spots in the cold, so keep them as warm and as *dry* as possible. If you find that your hands get too warm and sweaty in heavy gloves, try thin ones made of the same fabrics that go into long underwear—polypropylene or capilene. If your feet get cold, try a thin polyester sock underneath a thicker, wool-blend sock. Lace your shoes a little

more loosely in the winter; this leaves room for warm air to circulate around your feet. Too snug a fit will also cut off the flow of blood to your feet, which makes them get cold.

- If a hat makes you too warm, try a headband to protect your ears. If wool makes your forehead itch, try fleece.
- If there's snow or ice on the ground, you need shoes that have some traction. Lightweight hiking boots may be better than walking shoes in winter.
- If it's windy on a cool day, try to start your walk by heading into the wind—that way you won't go too far with the wind at your back, only to realize it's freezing cold when you turn around.
- Finally, don't forget fluids. You still need to transport nutrients and oxygen—and especially heat—around your body when it's cold outside. If cold water doesn't sound appealing, try some herbal tea before and after a walk.

MUSIC: WALKING IN RHYTHM

Music really helps me get revved up on a walk. I know which tunes are at the right speed to keep my pace up, and I let the rhythm drive my feet. You may choose to walk to the tunes you like best, but why not put music to work for you by selecting songs with rhythm—in beats per minute—that corresponds to your footfalls? That way, you keep up your speed by keeping pace with the music.

The easiest way to do this is to use one of the walking audiotapes on the market. My WALKFIT tape includes music with the appropriate beats per minute for Foundation and Workout walks, along with some coaching from me along the way.

You can also make your own walking tape. Figure out

a song's beats per minute the same way you figure out your heart rate: Count the beats for 10 seconds, then multiply by 6. Then match beats per minute with the paces in the WALKFIT program. For Foundation and warm-up: 114 to 120 beats per minute. For Workout: 126 to 132 beats per minute. For intervals: 138 beats per minute or more.

There was an interesting study a couple of years ago, in which researchers found that people were able to keep exercising longer when they listened to music. The funny thing was that softer, slower "easy listening" music seemed to keep people going longer than loud, fast rock tunes. The researchers speculated that maybe quieter music keeps you more relaxed, so that you exercise more efficiently. Still, there's no right or wrong kind of music: Whatever gets *you* going is what's best for you.

SAFETY ON THE STREET

Sometimes it's tempting to shut off your brain when you go out for a walk: Just turn off all that noise (or turn up the volume) and shift into cruise control for an hour. While I think it's important to clear your head during a walk, you do need to keep your wits about you. Walkers are most vulnerable to danger from cars, but crime is also a concern, particularly for women walking alone. A few tips for staying safe:

• If you're walking on a road, walk into traffic. That way, you can see vehicles coming at you and move out of their way.

• If you walk before sunrise or after sunset, wear reflective gear. Sporting goods and running specialty stores sell reflective vests and reflective bands that go around your ankles; some jogging suits come with reflective panels, and some walking shoes have reflective trim.

• If you use a personal stereo, keep one earpiece off so you can pick up sounds from the world around you. This is obviously important when you're walking near cars and traffic, but it's also a good practice on a sidewalk or multi-use pathway. That way, you can hear the bicyclist or skater yelling, "On your right!" just before they whiz by you at 15 miles an hour.

• You're always safer walking with another person, or with a dog, than you are walking alone. If you're going to walk by yourself, use good judgment: Avoid isolated areas, and consider carrying a whistle or noisemaker.

5

≣

Walking Away
from Fat

Jeopardy contestant #1: I'll take "Health" for $1000, Alex.
Alex Trebek: These compounds—also known as glycerides—
   are the source of most Americans' weight problems.
Contestant #1: What are sugars, Alex?
Buzzzz.
Alex: No, that's not it.
Contestant #2: What are *fats*, Alex?
Ding, ding, ding.
Alex: That's correct.

I don't mean to be glib, but it's really as simple as that.
One in four American adults—48 million people—are
dieting at any given time, wondering, "Why can't I lose
weight and keep it off?" The answer is fat: oils, butter,
fatty meats, mayonnaise, cheese, nuts. Fat, in all its guises,
is a root cause of weight problems. It's also a major cause
of health problems like heart disease and certain cancers.
Once you grasp this essential truth—and learn to control
fat in your diet—you're on your way to long-term weight
loss and better health.

More than 40 percent of the calories in the average American's diet come from fat. The United States Government and
the American Heart Association recommend a diet that's less
than 30 percent fat, and even this is for people who are

already at a healthy weight. For weight loss, most experts recommend a diet closer to 20 percent fat.

Health authorities recommend this amount of fat not because they want you to look better in a bathing suit, but because reducing the amount of fat in your diet reduces your risk factors for most of the diseases that Americans die from—heart disease, hypertension, diabetes, and certain kinds of cancer. In fact, even if you never reach what you think is an "ideal" weight (which may have more to do with a bathing suit than it does with your health), you will be a lot better off if you eat less fat.

A BAD FAT DAY

To get a real sense of how fat sneaks into your diet, let's take a look at an apparently "healthy" day of eating, bearing in mind that a 5'6" woman who wants to eat a 20 percent fat diet should consume only 33 grams of fat in a day. (There are charts for this later in the chapter.)

Let's start with our average woman's breakfast. She's read enough about cholesterol and fat by now that she's given up bacon and eggs (about 20 grams of fat in a two-slice, two-egg breakfast; 30 grams if you add two slices of buttered toast). Instead, she has:

• A small bran muffin with a pat of butter: 14 grams of fat
• Coffee with half-and-half: 2 grams of fat

Her "light" breakfast has 16 grams of fat, almost as much as the bacon and eggs. It's 9 a.m., and she's halfway to 33 grams of fat.

A mid-morning snack:

• "Just one" cookie: 3 grams

- A cup of coffee with one liquid nondairy creamer: 2 grams
- *Total: 5 grams*

On to a "light" lunch:

- A slice of bread with a pat of butter: 4 grams
- A large salad with two tablespoons of dressing: 14 grams
- Or a turkey sandwich with mayonnaise: 18 grams
- *Total: 18 grams*

This brings her day's total to 39 grams of fat, which means she's already 6 grams over the top, with her main meal still ahead of her.

But first, an afternoon snack:

- A handful of nuts and raisins, 10 grams
- *Total: 10 grams*

And, finally, dinner:

- A small steak: 9 grams (if she trimmed the visible fat)
- A baked potato with 2 tablespoons of sour cream: 5 grams
- Vegetables, with 1/4 cup of cheese sauce: 8 grams
- She skips dessert because she's watching her weight.
- *Total: 22 grams*

Day's Total: 71 grams of fat. That's more than twice the recommended amount. Despite this woman's best intentions, this was a 41 percent fat day, "average" for an American. Notice there was no ice cream sundae, no fudge brownie, and no fried food, and that the meals were of modest size and nutritionally balanced. But small amounts of fats, which she probably ate without a moment's thought, turned a healthy diet into a weight problem.

Why? Because a gram of fat contains 9 calories. A gram of carbohydrate or protein contains 4 calories. Same weight, twice the calories. That's why one level tablespoon of oil, a tiny drizzle, has 120 calories, more than a large banana.

It would have been easy to cut out much of that 71 grams of fat with some simple substitutions, like:

- putting low-fat milk in coffee
- topping the baked potato with low-fat yogurt or cottage cheese
- replacing the mayonnaise on the sandwich with mustard
- substituting fat-free salad dressing
- having a low-fat snack like pretzels instead of nuts and raisins

That's a savings of almost 30 grams of fat right there, and we haven't even attacked the butter yet! And none of these changes involves eating any less food.

Which is why, if you want to lose weight and keep it off, you have to reduce the amount of fat in your diet—maybe drastically. That's what it all boils down to, all the diet plans, books, and magazine articles with promise-the-world titles like "Eat everything in sight and be light as a feather": Cut out the fat.

Some people do have genetic predispositions to obesity that may make it harder for them to reach an "ideal" weight. But obese people can still lose weight and become significantly more healthy by exercising and eating less fat.

YOUR FAT BUDGET

So how do you get down to a 20 percent fat diet? You can start by cutting out added fats, like salad dressing, creamy sauces, whole-milk dairy products, and fatty meats, and replacing them with sensible substitutions. We'll get into these later.

But it's not enough just to say, "Cut out the fat." Fats are far too common and far too slippery for that. You're going to have to be vigilant about it, at least at first. To rein in fat consumption, you have to closely monitor your fat intake. The simplest way to do that is to count the grams of fat that you eat.

A diet that's 20 percent fat actually translates to a certain number of grams of fat per day, depending on your height and gender. Using the Fat Budget charts (see pp. 71 and 72), find your height and gender, and you'll see how many grams of fat add up to a 20 percent fat diet for you. For instance, as a 5'8" woman, I get a budget of 35 grams of fat per day. I can use them however I wish, but that's all I get.

Your fat budget is now your magic number: two digits that will change your life. Throughout the day, keep track of what you eat and the number of fat grams the foods contain. (Later I'll explain how to use a daily diary to keep track of food choices and fat grams.) When you reach the magic number, you've used up your allotment—that's it for fat for the day.

This method works because it forces you to be conscious of what you're eating. When you start counting fat grams, you'll learn where fat lurks and how quickly it adds up. Of course, sometimes the truth hurts: Maybe you've suspected all along that those two slices of cheese on your sandwich were a bad idea. But you never guessed that two little slices of cheese add 18 grams of fat—half your fat budget!

At some point, if you're serious about losing weight you're going to have to face the music: Nowhere in the Constitution does it guarantee your right to two slices of cheese on your sandwich and a piece of pie for dessert.

Fat Budget for Men

Height (without shoes)	20% Fat Budget
	Per Day Grams
5'1"	33
5'2"	33
5'3"	34
5'4"	35
5'5"	36
5'6"	37
5'7"	38
5'8"	39
5'9"	41
5'10"	42
5'11"	43
6'	44
6'1"	45
6'2"	47
6'3"	48
6'4"	49

WHERE'S THE FAT?

Now start reading labels! Because of the government's new food-labeling laws, you can look at a label and see the total number of grams of fat per serving. (The label will also tell you the percentage of the day's total fat calories that the food contains, but this number is based on a 30 percent fat diet, so it doesn't apply to us.) The label also tells you the number of grams of each kind of fat—saturated, polyunsaturated, and monounsaturated. This is useful, since you want to keep saturated fats to a minimum (more about that later), but you still have to count the *total number* of grams of fat.

Fat Budget for Women

Height (without shoes)	20% Fat Budget
	Per Day Grams
4'8"	25
4'9"	26
4'10"	26
4'11"	27
5'	28
5'1"	29
5'2"	29
5'3"	30
5'4"	31
5'5"	32
5'6"	33
5'7"	34
5'8"	35
5'9"	36
5'10"	37
5'11"	39
6'	40
6'1"	41
6'2"	42

Meats are also subject to new labeling laws: If meat, fish, or poultry is advertised as lean, it must contain less than 10 grams of fat, and less than 4 grams of saturated fat per 3-ounce serving. To be extra lean, a serving must have fewer than 5 grams of total fat, and 2 grams of saturated fat or less.

For the fat content of unpackaged foods, you'll need a pocket-sized fat-gram book. These are easy to find at bookstores.

SIZING UP PORTIONS

At the same time, start educating yourself about serving sizes. If you don't already have a small kitchen scale, I recommend getting one. They only cost a few dollars, and, for weight-loss purposes they'll do you a lot more good than the scale in your bathroom.

Now start sizing up portions. Weigh out 2.5 ounces of chicken, then compare that to the amount of meat that comes on a dinner plate at a restaurant. Weigh out 3 ounces of sliced meat, and compare that to the amount that comes on a deli sandwich. Weigh the muffin that you get at the bakery: If a 3-ounce muffin has 10 grams of fat, and your muffin weighs 6 ounces . . . uh-oh.

Measure out a measly little tablespoon of oil and pour it on a plate: There's 13 grams of fat! Take a look at a level tablespoon of sour cream or cheese sauce—it's not much. Figure out how much half-and-half you dump in your coffee. This will really drive home just how fast those fat grams add up.

With packaged foods, always check the serving size on the label: If a box of cereal says it has 1 gram of fat per 1-ounce serving, and (like most people) you put closer to 2 ounces of cereal in your bowl, you have to count 2 grams of fat.

If all this measuring sounds a little neurotic, don't worry: You're not going to have to do it for the rest of your life. Once you've spent some time getting familiar with portions, you'll be able to eyeball things realistically. Instead of saying, "I just had a little cheese sauce on my vegetables," you'll know that it was more like 4 tablespoons—and that's half your fat for the day.

"BANKING" FAT GRAMS

Counting fat grams means that you don't have to rule out any foods. If you're really dying for a high-fat treat, you can have it, as long as you stay within your budget. I don't recommend spending all your fat grams on ice cream every day—it's not a nutritious way to eat—but there's nothing wrong with eating what you love now and then.

I will sometimes "bank" fat grams over a two-day period: If I know I'm eating out Thursday night, I'll cut back on my fat grams on Wednesday. I'll still stick to the healthier foods on the menu—say, grilled chicken or fish, or a pasta dish without cream sauce—but if I've banked an extra 10 grams, I don't have to worry about large restaurant portions, or I can treat myself to dessert.

Don't let banking turn into a cycle of depriving yourself and then bingeing. Try to stick to your budget most of the time.

BASIC DAILY MEAL PLAN FOR WEIGHT LOSS

Counting fat grams is the best way to get your fat intake under control, and reducing the fat in your diet is the first step to healthier eating. Now let's build on that good start with a well-balanced plan for healthy eating and weight loss.

With the following basic daily meal plan, you can choose from a variety of foods to create a filling, nutrient-rich, high-energy diet. If you stick to these guidelines, you should find it easy to stay within your fat budget. Your fat budget will also steer you to lower-fat choices within each of the food groups.

Three Big Fat Myths

While we're on the subject of fat, let's clear up some common misconceptions.

Q. If less fat is better, isn't no fat best of all?

A. No. While fat is public enemy #1, we do need some of it in our diet. Our bodies use fatty acids for growth and repair, and fat helps us absorb important fat-soluble vitamins like A, D, E, and K. Small amounts of fat also help with weight control, since meals containing some fat take longer to digest, so you feel full longer. Finally, of course, fat tastes good. Its molecular structure is designed to make your tongue happy, and struggling against that basic truth can drive you crazy.

Q. Aren't monounsaturated fats good for you?

A. Yes and no. The first thing to look at is your *total* fat consumption. If it's too high, it doesn't matter what kind of fats you're eating: Too much fat is bad. Once you reduce the *total* fat in your diet, it is true that polyunsaturated and monounsaturated fats are preferable to saturated fats. Saturated fats are the worst offenders when it comes to raising cholesterol levels, a major risk factor for heart disease. That's why the U.S. Government and the American Heart Association recommend getting less than 10 percent of your daily calories from saturated fats.

Monounsaturated fats: olive oil, canola oil, avocado
Polyunsaturated fats: vegetable oils, nuts and seeds

Saturated fats: whole-milk dairy products, meats, tropical oils (coconut, cocoa butter, palm oil)

Q. For heart disease, isn't it more important to cut out cholesterol?

A. Not necessarily. Both the cholesterol and saturated fat in food can increase your blood cholesterol levels, and in most people's diets, saturated fats are the bigger problem. It's important to limit your intake of high-cholesterol foods: Animal products like egg yolks and organ meats contain the most. But the "no cholesterol" claims on the packages of many fattening foods can be *very* misleading: A cookie made with palm kernel oil (not an animal product, but high in saturated fat) may not *contain* cholesterol, but it will still increase your blood cholesterol level.

This plan is not about counting calories. However, using the recommended number of servings from the various food groups, women will eat about 1,200 calories per day, and men will get 1,500 calories. Later, in the maintenance phase, you'll increase your daily calories by adding more servings.

Basic Daily Meal Plan

Your meals should include:

For Women	For Men
2 milk servings	2 milk servings
3 or more vegetable servings	3 or more vegetable servings
2–3 fruit servings	3 fruit servings

5 starch servings   6 starch servings
5 ounces of meat   6 ounces of meat

Starch Group

For a long time, people thought that starchy foods like pasta, bread, and potatoes made you fat. I'm absolutely amazed that I *still* hear people worrying that they shouldn't be eating bread or pasta because they're trying to lose weight. Filling, nutritious, high in fiber, and nonfattening, carbohydrates are high-octane fuel for your body. They should make up the bulk of your diet.

To increase the amount of fiber in your diet, shop for whole-grain breads and grains: couscous, brown or wild rice, bread made from whole or cracked wheat (not "unbleached wheat flour") and high-fiber cereals—compare labels. Potatoes are high in fiber only if you eat the skin.

The trouble with starches is the high-fat toppings we pour all over them. For low-fat toppings, try yogurt, cottage cheese, or salsa on a potato. Stick to red sauces for pasta (you can make your own without added oil), and avoid pesto and cream sauces. For bread, make yogurt cheese, a cream cheese substitute. Just put nonfat yogurt in cheesecloth and leave it overnight in your refrigerator. The water drips out, leaving a spreadable cheese.

A serving of starch is a piece of bread or half a muffin or bagel; 1/2 cup of pasta, rice, or cooked cereal; a small baked potato; an ounce of dry cereal; a tortilla, small roll, or small muffin; an ounce of crackers. Beans are high in protein and fiber, 1/3 cup of cooked beans or peas is a high-protein, high-fiber serving of starch.

Vegetable Group

Vegetables are also high in fiber and carbohydrates. They also happen to be packed with important nutrients, vitamins like A, C, and beta-carotene, which have been linked to reduced rates of cancer and heart disease.

Vegetables aren't just for dinner! Eat them at lunch, and as snacks. Carrots, steamed green beans, celery, and peppers all make great, portable, vitamin-rich snacks. Most vegetables are high in fiber, and the cruciferous vegetables—broccoli, cauliflower, brussel sprouts, and kale—are very high in vitamins and minerals.

One serving is 1 cup of raw leafy vegetables, or 1/2 cup of other vegetables.

Fruit Group

Fruits make great snacks and great desserts. Citrus fruits are packed with fiber and nutrients; fruits with edible skin tend to have a little more fiber. To make fruit more of a treat, make a dessert plate with small amounts of several kinds of fruits—sliced melon, berries, and grapes, for example.

A serving is 1 medium-size piece of fruit, 1/2 cup of cooked or canned fruit or 1/4 cup of dried fruit, or 1/2 cup of fruit juice. With certain high-calorie fruits—grapes and cherries, for example—it's best to eat smaller portions. Bananas are very nutritious and filling, but keep in mind that they have almost twice the calories per serving of other fruits. Limit them to one a day.

Milk Group

Switch to nonfat or low-fat dairy products. If you don't like the taste of nonfat dairy products, most markets now carry 1% fat milk, yogurt, and cottage cheese. Low-fat cheeses are also available, but these are still much higher in fat than low-fat yogurt or cottage cheese, so stick to 1-ounce portions.

Sugar-free, low-fat hot chocolate and shakes are tasty alternatives. Low-fat frozen yogurt, while low in fat, is usually high in calories and has only half the nutrients found in regular yogurt, so think of it as a treat, not a dairy serving.

A milk serving is 1 ounce of cheese (2 tablespoons of parmesan or romano cheese), 2 tablespoons of cream cheese, 1/2 cup of cottage cheese, 1/4 cup of ricotta cheese, a cup of milk, or a cup of yogurt.

Meat Group

Your body uses protein for muscle building and repair, but you probably get more than you need every day. The average American diet is not only too high in fat, it's unnecessarily high in protein as well. There's a connection: The most common sources of protein are meat and dairy products, which are also high in fat.

In addition to getting most of our protein from fatty foods, we tend to eat it in portions that are too large. A couple of 2.5-ounce servings of meat provide all the protein you need in a day, but a typical single serving of meat—a hamburger, deli sandwich, or chicken breast—is more like 4 to 6 ounces. Weigh it out and see for yourself.

Here's where you can trim a lot of fat out of your diet, literally. By eating smaller portions of lean meat—fish, poultry without the skin, lean pork or beef with all visible fat trimmed off—you can save a huge number of calories and fat grams. Trim the fat or remove the skin before cooking meat and poultry.

In this meal plan, a serving of meat is generally 2.5 to 3 ounces.

Water

Water is the simplest and most powerful element of good nutrition. Our bodies need water to perform almost every vital metabolic function. Dehydration is a real energy zapper: Often when you feel tired late in the day it's because you're slightly dehydrated. (If you then seek a boost from a cup of coffee, which is a diuretic, the problem only worsens.) Dehydration can cause headaches as well.

Water also helps with weight control: A glass of water before meals can help fill you up, and drinking with meals can slow down a fast eater. Drinking throughout the day keeps your energy up, so you don't feel the need for that late-afternoon candy bar. Finally, if you're increasing the insoluble fiber in your diet, it's important to drink plenty of water to avoid constipation

Drink at least *eight glasses of water* each day. It takes a little effort to drink that much, but I find that it makes a huge difference. For variety, try flavored seltzer and mineral waters, and hot or iced herbal teas. Or splash a little fruit juice in your bubbly water or tea. No-calorie beverages are an easy way to eliminate calories from your diet, so choose them over sodas and juices. Diet sodas are OK, but water and tea are healthier choices.

About Combination Foods

Some dishes, like pizza or salad plates, contain foods from several groups. When eating such dishes, just estimate which groups and, more importantly, how many servings of each they include.

WHAT'S NOT HERE

Notice that I'm not telling you what *not* to eat. Your fat budget will get rid of most of that—fried foods, whole-fat dairy, mayonnaise, fatty cuts of meat.

What about sugar? Unless you are diabetic, sugar actually isn't "bad for you"; it doesn't promote any diseases except tooth decay. The problem is that most sweet treats like ice cream and candy bars are full of fat. Other sweets that don't contain fats, like soda, syrup, and jam, have no real nutritional value, but they do have plenty of calories. Use them sparingly, but if it's a choice between jam and butter on your toast, go for the jam.

MAKING IT WORK

In Chapter 2, I talked about changing habits, and how important it is to apply some mind power to the task. The four-part strategy I outlined in that chapter is equally useful here:

Breaking down mental barriers
Establishing specific, inspirational goals
Making a plan you can live with
Making a commitment to your plan

If you need to, go back and read Chapter 2 again, especially the section "Breaking Down Barriers."

With weight loss, you have to set small, specific, attainable goals. You can't change a lifetime's worth of tastes and habits in a week. If you're used to eating four servings from the milk group each day, and you need to reduce that to two servings, you may want to try three servings a day for a few weeks as an intermediate step. If you eat a 40 percent fat diet, it may take some time before you can comfortably manage on a 20 percent fat budget. Cut out fat grams gradually, if you need to, but cut them.

Instead of setting goals in terms of pounds lost, define your goals in terms of changing habits. Rather than trying to lose two pounds this week, make a goal of adding more vegetables to your diet or getting in the habit of eating smaller portions of meat.

Daily Diary

A daily diary is a great way to make an eating plan and to monitor your commitment to that plan. In the beginning, it will also help you get a clear picture of how you eat now. By writing down *everything,* you'll begin to see when and why you get into trouble.

In your daily food diary, record the following:

1. The time of your meal or snack, and how long it took you to eat it.
2. What you ate. Be specific: "6 ounces of yogurt," not just "yogurt." Or "20 tortilla chips," instead of "chips."
3. The number of grams of fat you ate.
4. Where you ate.
5. Any thoughts associated with eating, such as, "I'm eating because I'm tired," or, "I didn't have time to fix something better."

Be thorough and honest in your diary. The point of keeping it is to figure out where things go wrong: Do you skip meals and end up hungry in a place where there are no good food choices? Do you eat more on days when you don't eat breakfast? Is there something that's consistently pushing you over your fat budget? Do you need a satis-fying, low-fat snack in the afternoon to stave off the predin-ner munchies?

Use the diary to start planning meals in advance. Put-ting menus down on paper is a good way to get used to the food group system. And just by taking the time to make entries in your diary or plan for the days ahead, you'll put more mental energy into problem solving.

Lose Some, Win Some

If you're consistently exercising, living within your fat bud-get, and following this eating plan, *you will lose weight*, but don't let the scale rule your life: Weigh yourself *no more than once a week*, on the same scale and at the same time of day. On average, you might lose between one-half pound and two pounds per week, but don't be thrown by plateaus or even slight increases, which are often just fluctuations in fluids.

Over a period of months, your weight will drop, but that shouldn't be your only measure of success. If your clothes fit better but you weigh the same amount, you've probably traded fat weight for lean muscle mass. You may also have more energy, or fewer headaches, or feel more in control of your life: Those gains are as meaningful as pounds lost!

Don't get hung up on a particular number of pounds that you think you need to lose. I've seen people lose 20 pounds, but instead of enjoying the fact that they look and feel better, they raise the stakes: "Now I just want to lose 15 more pounds. *Then* I'll be happy." But they don't have enough motivation to stick with it for another 15 pounds, and they quickly get frustrated.

If after losing weight you reach a plateau, and you start

to feel defeated, stop pushing yourself. Instead of trying to lose more, focus on what you've already accomplished and put your energy into maintenance. It's more important to keep off what you've lost, and to get used to the idea that exercise and low-fat eating are lifelong habits. You may be able to lose more weight later on, or you may realize that you're fine as you are.

MAINTENANCE

Once you've reached your weight-loss goal—or if you want to take a break from trying to lose weight but don't want to lose ground—shift to a maintenance program that's slightly higher in calories. As long as you keep walking and continue to keep your fat grams down around 20 percent, you won't gain back any weight.

To figure out your maintenance-level plan, get your approximate daily calorie needs by multiplying your weight by 15. (You would multiply by 13 if you were sedentary, but you're going to be walking—right?) Then use the basic daily maintenance plan that's closest to your total. For example, I weigh 130 pounds. I multiply that by 15 and get 1,950 calories. That puts me closest to the 2,000-calorie plan.

Calories	Milk		Vegetable		Fruit		Starch		Meat
1,200	2 servings		3 servings		2 servings		5 servings		5 oz.
1,500	2	"	3	"	2	"	6	"	6 oz.
1,800	2	"	3	"	3	"	7	"	8 oz.
2,000	2	"	4	"	4	"	8	"	8 oz.
2,200	3	"	4	"	5	"	9	"	8 oz.

A HEALTHY CYCLE

If you're trying to lose weight, there are two simple things to learn from this book: 1) Walk regularly, and 2) Learn to find fat, count it, and cut it out of your life.

This is not a quick-weight-loss plan. It's not even a "diet." It's a strategy for changing the way you eat so that you will lose excess weight now and control your weight for the rest of your life. Too often, people approach weight loss thinking, "I'm going to stick with this until I lose twenty-five pounds . . ." But then what? Do you go back to the eating habits that got you into the trouble in the first place?

Fat is like the weeds in a garden: You can pull out all the weeds, but if you leave the roots in the ground, they'll grow back in no time. Well, you can go on "a diet" to get rid of excess weight, but if you don't get to the root of the problem by changing your habits, the fat will come back. By learning about fat—how much you should be eating, where it hides, and how to avoid it—you are successfully pulling those roots.

When you switch to a healthier way of eating, not only will you lose weight and keep it off, but you'll get other benefits as well. People tell me that they feel better about themselves, that their skin and hair looks healthier, and that their backaches and headaches go away. Healthy food gives you more energy day in and day out. In fact, eating well and exercising create a positive cycle: When you eat well and exercise, you start to lose weight and gain energy. Exercise gets easier, and so does weight loss.

I love to tell the story of Peggy and Brent Suddick, of Omaha, Nebraska, a couple I met at a walking event in San Francisco. Peggy, age 27, and Brent, 32, were faithful about WALKFIT and cut most of the fat out of their diets. As a result they each lost about 40 pounds last year. While Brent and Peggy felt great about how they looked and were enjoying being in the best shape of their lives, they seemed most proud of the fact that they had successfully changed their lifestyle:

"I don't call this 'a diet,' " says Peggy. "We're eating healthy now. Before, high-fat foods were our favorites."

"We'd have BLTs for lunch every day," laughs Brent.

"And lots of cheese," says Peggy. "But now, we eat low-fat cheese, and it tastes creamy and good like whole cheese would."

"And low-fat dressing," adds Brent. "You can't even tell the difference."

Brent loves to go to the supermarket and read labels now. He jokes about how so many labels say they only have 1 gram of fat per serving—"and then you look at how much a serving is, and you realize you would eat ten times that much."

Peggy and Brent thought they would feel deprived when they cut the fat out of their diets, but they really haven't. But what pleases them most is the fact that their three-year-old son, Marshall, is growing up eating healthy food, not "the cupcake and cookie diet," says Dad. Marshall loves all kinds of fruit, his mom reports, and he's keeping an open mind about vegetables. "He likes carrots," says Peggy.

"Just the other day I was walking into the store with him," says Brent, "and he said, 'Daddy, when I'm bigger and a daddy, I'm going to like peppers and tomatoes, too.' "

Amazing.

Five Easy Steps to Better Eating

If you're not ready to adopt a whole new basic daily menu, but you do want to eat better, here are the five most important changes you can make, in addition to getting on a fat budget.

1. The simplest single way to improve your diet is to meet the U.S. Department of Agriculture's Food Pyramid recommendation of five servings of fruits and vegetables a day. Fruits and vegetables are low in fat, high in carbohydrates and fiber, and rich in important nutrients like beta-carotene and vitamin C. By eating five servings of fruits and veggies, you'll probably skip other, less-healthful foods. Think of vegetables at lunch and snack times—carrots, celery, pepper strips, for example—and fruits for dessert.

2. No *added* fats. Live within your fat budget by cutting out the most obvious sources of fat: whole-milk dairy products, butter, cheese, and meats. Choose low- or nonfat dairy, and eat small portions of lean meat from which all visible fat has been trimmed before cooking. Choose low-fat salad dressings and toppings for starches; in cooking, saute in wine or broth instead of butter and oil.

3. Drink water—eight or more glasses a day to keep energy up and appetite down. Try flavored sparkling waters, iced herbal teas, and plain old iced H_2O with a slice of lemon, lime, or orange, or with a mint leaf floating in it.

4. Eat regular meals, including breakfast. Overeating, out-of-control snacking, and poor food choices are more likely when you don't eat well at meals or skip meals altogether. Then you get very hungry, often when your choices are limited to bad or worse. As for breakfast, even a small one—a toasted bagel or yogurt

and fruit—will rev up your metabolic rate in the morning, so you'll burn more calories all day.

5. Eat a variety of foods, including lots of fruits and vegetables, whole-grain breads and cereals, low-fat dairy and protein. The carbohydrates on your plate—the fruits, vegetables, and starches—should occupy roughly twice as much space as the fats and proteins.

6

Walking Through Pregnancy

If it weren't for my first pregnancy, I don't know if I ever would have gotten hooked on walking. And if it weren't for walking, I don't know how I would have gotten through either of my pregnancies!

Back in 1988, when I was pregnant with Katie, my first, I kept up my normal workouts and activities for about four months. That included taking occasional weekend hikes with Steve. Around the fifth month, though, fighting gravity got more difficult, and when it got to the point where Steve was literally pushing me up the steep sections of the trail, we decided we'd had enough.

That was about the time that we started walking. At least three days a week, Steve and I would do a round-trip jaunt from our house to Westwood—about 3 miles. As I got bigger, we walked a little slower, and toward the end we'd walk the first mile and half, stop and have a bit to eat, and then walk home.

A week after Katie was born—8 pounds, 7 ounces; a normal delivery—I was out walking again. Soon I was taking her with me, carrying her in a pack on my chest. It felt great to be outdoors, and it was also a way to ease myself back into the routine of things but still be with Katie.

As I got back into shape, walking faster and harder, I realized that my body felt really good. At that point, instead of going back to my pre-pregnancy workout routine, I decided to learn more about walking. I started challenging myself with faster paces and longer distances. When Katie got older, I just put her in the baby jogger and kept on walking.

Two years after Katie's birth, I was pregnant again, and I walked right through *that* pregnancy. That's how Katie and Perrie, now five and two, have kept me focused on walking for the past five years. And having grown up with walking, they're starting to make it their own thing.

There's a park that's a 25-minute walk away from our house. It seems that every other day the girls want to go to the park. I always ask them if they want to drive or walk there, and at least half the time they want to walk. Even Perrie, who's only two, wants to walk the whole way.

So we pack up some snacks and some park toys, and we head out. Along the way we pass the toy store man, and our favorite frozen yogurt man, and the girls stop and say their friendly howdy-do's to everyone. Once we've exhausted all the swings and jungle gyms at the park, we wander home.

It really thrills me that my daughters have somehow "inherited" my love for walking; that what started in my first pregnancy has developed into a fun and healthy part of our family. My hope is that the information in this chapter will help make walking a healthy part of your family's life, too.

CHANGING ATTITUDES

For far too long, doctors were extremely conservative about the amount and kinds of physical activity that they recommended for pregnant women. Today, finally, most experts are convinced—mainly by evidence from women who refused to stop being active—that regular, moderate exercise is healthy for pregnant women.

In fact, the attitude within the medical world has shifted 180 degrees, from emphasizing the *bad* things that might happen if you exercise to pointing out what *good* things exercise does. Raul Artal, M.D., is the author of the book *Pregnancy and Exercise*. Dr. Artal guided me through my first pregnancy and helped me with my pregnancy videotape. According to his book, there are many ways in which exercise can enhance your pregnancy, and my own experience affirms this. These benefits include:

1. A more comfortable pregnancy.
2. Enhanced cardiovascular fitness and endurance. This means better delivery of oxygen and other nutrients throughout your body, which makes you feel more energetic.
3. Prevention or reduction of leg problems like varicose veins, cramps, and thrombosis (blood clotting).
4. Better muscle tone and strength, which makes it easier to carry that extra weight around and prepares you for toting a baby and a diaper bag.
5. Improved balance and coordination, which can be a problem for some pregnant women.
6. A better emotional state, which may help you deal with all the changes and challenges of pregnancy.

7. An easier return to your pre-pregnancy weight and fitness level.

Some experts also think that regular exercise may prevent or help manage gestational diabetes, a condition in which women become diabetic during pregnancy. This complication affects about 3 percent of pregnant women, but it has serious long-term consequences: Of women who get gestational diabetes, half will develop diabetes later in life.

There are still some lingering safety concerns. Doctors worry that certain kinds of exercise might have some risks for a pregnant woman or her fetus, and they still recommend avoiding jarring activities, vigorous exercise that produces a high heart rate or high body temperature, and exercise that involves sudden movements or deep-joint flexion or extension.

That's why walking is such a perfect exercise for pregnant women: It gives you all the benefits of exercise with none of the risks. Any active woman should consider walking through her pregnancy, but walking is so safe that an inactive woman can even *start* a program when she's pregnant. And with a normal pregnancy, you can walk regularly right up to the end, and pick it up again soon after a normal delivery.

Judy Mahle Lutter is president of the Melpomene Institute, a nonprofit organization devoted to research and education on women's health and fitness. Melpomene has done a lot of research on exercise and pregnancy. I first heard about Judy Lutter and Melpomene at a Women's Sports Foundation banquet in 1993, when Judy received the Foundation's Billie Jean King Contribution Award. When I picked up Melpomene's book *Bodywise Woman*, I knew I wanted to turn to Judy for her expertise on walking and pregnancy.

"Lots of women call Melpomene early in their pregnancy to find out what is appropriate, because this is a time when they start taking better care of themselves," says Lutter. "One of the things we suggest is that they start walking, particularly if they haven't been active," she says. "And when women call because they're finding that other activities are uncomfortable, we tell *them* to consider walking, too."

SPECIAL CONSIDERATIONS

Most women can be completely comfortable with the knowledge that walking is good for you and safe for your baby. It's still a good idea to talk to your obstetrician or midwife about exercise, since some circumstances do require caution, like a history of miscarriage, or multiple pregnancy, premature dilation, and other complications.

Even if you have an uncomplicated pregnancy, your body is in a special state. It won't perform as it normally does. It has new limits, and it needs some special care. Your heart and lungs, for example, work overtime during pregnancy just to supply oxygen to you and your developing fetus. If you try to exercise very hard, you'll quickly realize that you don't have much cardiovascular capacity left over; in other words, you'll be wheezing in no time. This is true even if you're very fit.

During pregnancy, it's more important than ever to listen to your body; if it's trying to tell you to cool it, do so. Here are a few other considerations for walking mothers-to-be:

Nutrition

Now is *not* the time to diet. It's very important to meet your growing body's daily calorie needs, and walking will increase those needs.

Ideally you want most of your calories to come from nutritious foods. Of course, during pregnancy it's sometimes difficult to be reasonable about food. In my case, after not having looked at a piece of bacon for about 15 years, I was possessed by the need to eat not one, not two, but *three* bacon, lettuce, and tomato sandwiches in a row. And after practically living on vegetables, I couldn't look at a vegetable for about three months. All I wanted was spicy food: Indian, Mexican, you name it—as spicy as could be.

So within the limits of your appetite, remember that low-fat foods are as healthy during pregnancy as at other times, as long as you're eating plenty of food. If you use pregnancy as an excuse to eat lots of fatty treats and sweets, you will probably gain both weight *and fat*.

"Gaining a healthy amount of weight is necessary for a healthy baby, but gaining fifty pounds will make it difficult to return to pre-pregnancy weight," explains Lutter. Eating well and exercising can help you minimize *excessive* weight gain.

Body Temperature

Most experts advise pregnant women not to get overheated, because of concerns about excessive body temperature and birth defects. With the following precautions, you can walk without worry:

• Stay well hydrated. Drink 16 ounces of water a half-hour before you start, and, if possible, a couple of sips every 15 minutes during your walk. You may want to walk somewhere with restrooms nearby, since you'll probably need to urinate frequently.
• Don't walk in high temperatures or high humidity.

- Don't walk if you have a fever.
- Wear cool, loose-fitting clothing to allow body heat to dissipate.
- Stop exercising if you feel that you're overheating.
- Avoid exercising when pollution levels are high—particularly at midday on hot, sunny days in urban areas. Pollutants like ozone aren't good for you, and they aren't good for the fetus, either.

Loose Joints

During pregnancy, hormonal changes make your connective tissues—tendons, cartilage, and ligaments—get softer. This is what eventually lets a baby's big head pass through a very small space, but in the time before and after your delivery it makes you injury-prone, because those tissues are easily strained.

Compared to many activities, walking is less likely to result in injury, but it's not completely without hazard. It's important not to overstride, which can put strain on your hip joint. Walk with your normal stride length, as you always should, and increase your pace by taking quicker steps. Any pre- or post-exercise stretching should be done slowly and gently.

Sports Bras

If you're normally small-breasted, you may not have much experience with sport bras. But starting in your second trimester, you may find that brisk walking hurts your breasts. That's the time to shop for a good, breathable, supportive sports bra. Several companies make sports bras especially for larger-breasted women. These usually have adjustable shoulder straps and clasps in the back for a perfect fit.

A good sports bra will also be a godsend after the birth, if you're planning to nurse. Otherwise, full breasts and exercise can be a painful combination.

THERE WILL BE DAYS . . .

I would be lying if I told you you're going to feel terrific all the time. There will be days, particularly in the first and last trimesters, when you'll feel like a slug. Don't get frustrated when you're low on energy. Your body is actually very, very busy; you just can't tell from the outside.

On days when you're lacking in spunk, try walking to see if it helps, but don't push yourself too hard. It's better not to set specific performance goals for yourself during pregnancy. Be flexible, and do the best you can day by day and month by month.

You can also expect to have some discomfort. A little achiness in your feet or legs is natural, and some women experience aches in the pelvic ligaments that are supporting the baby.

As your belly gets bigger, your center of gravity moves forward, and your back may begin to arch to compensate for the shift. This, combined with loosened connective tissue, results in back pain for about 50 percent of pregnant women. Melpomene Institute research found this to be equally true for exercising and nonexercising women. If you experience back pain, it makes sense to experiment in order to find out whether walking makes you feel better or worse.

These are all normal discomforts, but it's important to distinguish between "garden variety" fatigue and achiness and more serious warning signs. Stop walking if you experience any of the following:

- vaginal bleeding
- abdominal pain
- rapid heart beat (above 140 beats per minute)
- chest pain
- severe breathlessness
- headache, dizziness, nausea, or overheating

MONITORING INTENSITY

The standard calculation for target heart rate (60 to 80 percent of your maximum heart rate, which is 220 minus your age) isn't valid during pregnancy, because you're not working with a "normal" cardiovascular system. There's 30 to 50 percent more blood in your body than there was before, so your heart is working harder even when you're at rest.

Forget the THR charts for a few months, and monitor your intensity in one of the following three ways:

- Let your comfort level be your guide, but always keep your heart rate below 140 beats per minute. To check it, simply take your pulse at your wrist or neck when you've reached your maximum level of effort. If you're at or near 140, you should slow down. Staying below 140 should not be difficult with this walking program.
- Rate of perceived exertion (RPE), which is explained in Chapter 3, works very well during pregnancy. Try to stay within the 12 to 14 range—"moderate" to "somewhat hard." Don't go above 14.
- Use the talk test, also explained in Chapter 3. If you can carry on a conversation during your walk, you're not overdoing it.

WORKOUT GUIDELINES

Pre-pregnancy

If you're not yet pregnant but are planning to be, regular walking offers you a number of benefits. First of all, it won't interfere with conception. Extremely strenuous training does cause some women to stop menstruating, but unless you're a competitive race walker, it's almost impossible that walking will affect your fertility. If you have had difficulty conceiving in the past, ask your doctor for an opinion about walking.

Getting into shape before you conceive means you start your pregnancy in a healthier state. By improving your cardiovascular and musculo-skeletal condition and conceiving at a healthy weight, you may reduce the risk of complications like musculo-skeletal pain and gestational diabetes, circulation problems like varicose veins, and extreme fatigue.

If you are not yet pregnant, you can follow the guidelines in Chapter 3.

First Trimester

Research has not found a link between exercise in the first three months of pregnancy and increased incidence of miscarriage. Nor is there evidence that exercise in the first trimester increases the chance of later complications or birth defects.

What you can do during this period depends both on your fitness level and your individual reaction to being pregnant. Some women really struggle with morning sickness and fatigue in the first trimester; others don't. "Don't give up if you're feeling bad," advises Judy Lutter. "Don't beat yourself up, but keep trying. That will make it easier to get going again when you feel better."

I found that on the days when I felt really wretched, if I could just get out of the house and around the block, it made me feel much, much better. Sometimes you just have to get past that initial feeling of "I don't feel good and I can't do this." Once you get outdoors and breathe some fresh air, there's a good chance that you'll feel like walking.

Fitness levels are a little more predictable:

• If you're already an active walker, you can continue with your regular program—to the extent that your body is willing—through your first trimester.

• If, prior to getting pregnant, you regularly took part in another kind of exercise—30 to 40 minutes of aerobic activity, at least three times per week—and you want to switch to walking now, start by reading Chapter 3. Learn the basics of good walking form, then begin with a Level II or III workout: 40 to 60 minutes in Foundation, at a pace between 15 and 20 minutes per mile. You can gradually increase your pace, as long as you stay within the intensity guidelines above. Again, keep in mind that it's better not to have fixed goals about exercise when you're pregnant: Let your body have an opinion on how much you're going to do each day.

• If you never got around to that pre-pregnancy conditioning, you can still start a walking program after conception. Start by talking to your obstetrician or midwife about exercise. If you get a green light, begin in Level I, walking at a natural pace for as long as you are comfortable, for up to 30 minutes. For healthy but previously inactive women, walking three to four times a week for 30 to 40 minutes will be plenty of activity.

Second Trimester

For some women, this is the most comfortable, energetic portion of their pregnancy. "Even if you weren't able to exercise in your first trimester, there's no reason not to try again in month four. You may find that it's easier now," says Lutter. Staying active helps time go faster in this period, which sometimes seems to drag on forever.

If you continue walking regularly, you should be able to hold steady for a while. Chances are high that somewhere around the fifth or sixth month you'll start to slow down. Don't fight it.

Third Trimester

If you haven't slowed down by now, you will soon. Expect to drop back a level or two in pace, and be prepared for those zero-energy days. Try going for a walk, just to see if you feel better once you get moving.

Lung capacity becomes a limiting factor late in your pregnancy. At a certain point, it just feels like you can't find a breath of air. I found that if I could get out and walk in the morning, expanding my lungs a little made it easier for me to breathe for the rest of the day.

Keep walking as many days a week as you like: in a normal pregnancy, staying active should not increase the chance of premature delivery. In my second pregnancy, I walked—not very fast, of course—right up to my delivery day. Steve joked that I would have walked to the hospital, if he'd let me.

Postpartum

For lots of women, the postpartum period is difficult: Life changes dramatically, you may not be sleeping regularly, and there may even be some hormonally mediated depression. "The 'postpartum blues' takes a lot of forms," says Lutter. "It doesn't always immediately follow delivery. It may be weeks later that you have a hard time. But no matter what you call it, or when it happens, a positive way to deal with it is to go for a walk."

You should be able to walk within a week of a normal delivery. Start with short, slow, outings; whatever you can manage. Even a short stroll—just getting some fresh air and moving your body—can improve your mood.

Obviously, just because you've delivered your baby doesn't mean that your body is back to normal. Your heart rate will stay elevated for up to a month, for example, and your joints will still be loose for a while. When you feel ready to start walking your way back into shape, begin in Level I or II, or wherever you left off at the end of your pregnancy. Increase the duration and speed of your walks *gradually*. According to Melpomene Institute surveys, it takes most active women six to nine months to get back to pre-pregnancy form.

Nursing mothers should be sure to drink a lot of water. You may also be more comfortable walking if you nurse right before you go out the door. Women who are breast feeding should not be surprised if their post-pregnancy weight loss is a little slower.

Of course, there are other new challenges now, like what to do with the baby while you walk. I find that it's easy to get back in shape with an infant, because you can just put the baby in a backpack or baby jogger. Combining kids and fitness gets tougher when there's more than one, or when they're too big to go in the baby jogger but not big enough to ride a bicycle alongside you. Ideally there's someone else—namely Dad or another relative—who can entertain the kids while you spend 40 minutes doing something that's very important to you.

JOY MONTARBO

Remember Joy Montarbo from Chapter 1? She's the woman from Vancouver, Washington, who had a hard time sticking with other kinds of exercise but got hooked on walking. Joy, who is 35, also happens to be the mother of five children, with one more on the way.

Joy started doing WALKFIT after the birth of her fifth, and with the combination of walking and a low-fat diet, she got back to her pre-pregnancy weight for the first time in eight years. She kept walking when she became pregnant with number six. In her sixth month, Joy was still walking 4 miles at a 15-minute-per-mile pace, four times a week.

"This is the first time that I've done any serious walking during a pregnancy," she says. "It definitely keeps my energy level higher. Some days I wake up tired, but if I go ahead and walk I feel more energetic afterward."

Joy noticed other changes as well. "With my last couple of pregnancies I developed varicose veins, but when I walk they don't hurt so much at the end of the day. When I skip a day of exercising, my legs really ache," she says. And, she adds, "So far, my weight gain has been less with this pregnancy, but the baby is growing the way it's supposed to. I think that's going to help me afterward."

How does Joy, with five young children and one on the way, find time to walk? "I used to depend on my husband to watch the kids when I went for a walk," she explains. "That didn't always work out, so I got a treadmill. Now I can walk whenever I feel like it, whether my husband is available or not."

ADDITIONAL RESOURCES

• Melpomene Institute's Pregnancy and Exercise packet. Available for $12 from the Melpomene Institute, 1010

University Avenue, St. Paul, MN 55104; (612) 642-1951.

- *Bodywise Woman,* Human Kinetics Press, 1993. Available in bookstores and from the Melpomene Institute.
- *Pregnancy and Exercise*, by Raul Artal and G. S. Sharpe, Delacorte Press, 1992.

7

Mixing It Up: Walking Workout Options

Every now and then, I make a point of mixing things up and trying out a new kind of workout. I'll go to a class I've never taken, like tai chi or boxing, or I'll go somewhere I've never been for a hike.

Some of these experiments are busts, of course, like the time I tried in-line skating and broke my ankle. No kidding. Steve is great on skates, so he wanted to get me on blades. I was planning to run a 10K the following day, and I just wanted to do something that wasn't too strenuous. I ended up in the hospital, having pins surgically placed in my tibia! Needless to say, I never made it to that 10K.

Usually, though, trying new things doesn't result in catastrophe, and occasionally I find something that I really enjoy. I don't experiment like this because I'm bored with my usual workouts. I do it for the excitement of a new experience, and for the opportunity to learn. It keeps me looking at exercise with a fresh eye. I even learned something when I broke my leg—how to get a great workout using only your upper body!

WALKFIT can be your springboard to all kinds of new, walking-related activities. Hiking, walking clubs, race walking, road races, and walk-jog workouts are just a few of the suggestions in this chapter for new directions in which you can wander.

These options can make it a lot easier to be consistent about exercise. That's because making a lifelong commitment to exercise is a lot like making a lifelong commitment to another person: You have to expect ups and downs, ebbs and flows in your enthusiasm. There will be times when getting outside and going for a walk is *exactly* what you want to be doing—no carrot dangling required. But now and then you may find that you need some fresh inspiration.

If you find yourself getting into a rut, try one of these suggestions for putting a new spin on your walks. In the long run, I think you'll find that fast walking, like a good relationship, is your "old reliable": It's always there, and you'll keep coming back to it.

HEAD FOR THE HILLS

"When we walk, we naturally go to the fields and woods: What would become of us if we walked only in a garden or in a mall?" Believe it or not, those words were written in the 1850s, by Henry David Thoreau. Although Thoreau had a different kind of mall in mind when he wrote this, his sentiment is even more appropriate now.

All my life, I've loved walking in fields and woods, only I've always called it hiking. In fact, the first time Steve asked me on a date, I suggested going for a hike. We went out to one of my favorite trails in the Santa Monica

Mountains, and when he was still with me after 40 minutes, I thought, "Hey, this guy's okay!" Steve still says it almost killed him.

As I got more and more into walking and learned to increase my pace, I realized that a hard, fast walk can challenge me in the same way hiking does, and can make my body feel just as good. And, not surprisingly, the more I walk the more hiking becomes a part of my life.

Now Steve and the girls and I are frequent visitors to the hiking trails in the Los Angeles basin, but we've also gone hiking on vacations to places like Wyoming, Montana, Colorado, and the Grand Canyon. One of Perrie's favorite vacation souvenirs is a picture from last summer of the four of us on a trail, with a family of elk running by.

Some of my most glorious days have been spent on the trail, hiking with Steve or with friends. Wherever I go for a hike, whether it's in the desert or the alpine forest, I get a sense of peace, of being liberated from pavement and cars and phones and TV. It's really more like play than exercise—like the kind of exploring we used to do as kids. Walking and a trail map are all you need to start exploring again.

Getting Started

The only real difference between a hike and a long walk is that the going is slower on a hilly, unpaved trail. You should have good endurance—and modest goals—when you head out for a hike. Prepare yourself with fitness walks of at least 90 minutes. If possible, find a walking route that includes inclines, and then work your way up to steeper hills.

Distances are deceiving on a hike. A 4-mile walk on level ground might be easy, but that can be a long way on the trail. I allow for a hiking speed of 1.5 to 2 miles per hour, compared to 4 MPH or better on pavement. That slower pace includes frequent rest breaks, which often come naturally as you stop to take a family portrait, with elk, or to admire a purple and gold wildflower carpet.

Hiking uphill is hard work. On a 10 percent grade—a trail that rises 10 feet for every 100 feet in length—your heart rate will be about 20 percent higher than it is on level ground. Depending on your weight, you'll also use 80 to 100 percent more calories per minute on the uphills. For example, a 130-pound person who burns 3.5 calories per minute on flat ground would burn 6 calories per minute on a 10 percent grade. On steep stuff, especially at high altitude, you may need to stop frequently to rest.

Your muscles—particularly your quadriceps (thighs), the gluteals in your butt, and your hip flexors—have to work very hard to overcome gravity. Even the fittest walker may feel some soreness in those muscles after a long day of hiking.

You would think that the payoff for climbing up is that you get to coast on the downhill. Unfortunately, descents are taxing, too. While a 10 percent uphill doubles your effort, a 10 percent descent requires almost the same energy as walking on level ground. The reason: Resisting gravity takes energy. With each downhill step, the full weight of your body must be caught and slowed. This braking action is also hard on your muscles and joints. If you have any old injuries in your ankles, knees, or back, you may feel some discomfort during downhills.

Slipping can be a problem on downhills, but you can minimize it by using good form: First, try not to lean or sit back into the hill. Then, tighten up your abdominals to shift your pelvis forward slightly. This will get more of your weight over your feet, which really increases traction. Don't fight gravity more than you have to. Let your speed naturally increase on downhills, as long as you don't get out of control. It's a good idea to rest and drink water on descents, even if you're not sweating or out of breath.

The net result of all this climbing and descending is excellent total fitness. From your ankles and calves to your abdominals and the stabilizing muscles of the pelvis and lower back, hiking is great conditioning. On the aerobic side, this type of low-intensity, long-duration workout is a great way to increase endurance. Over hilly terrain, you'll get an interval workout, with intermittent periods of higher-intensity effort, to boost caloric expenditure and increase your maximum aerobic capacity.

Your body is working hard, so be good to it. Snack when you feel like it, and drink plenty of water. While you might not always take water with you on a walk, it's a must on a hike. Hiking uses a lot of energy, and there are no water fountains out there.

Be especially careful if you're hiking in hot weather, or at altitudes of over 4,000 feet. You're likely to get more tired in the thin air, and dehydration strikes quickly up high. Exhaustion, dizziness, nausea, headache, and confusion are all warning signs of heat exhaustion.

Finding Your Way

A hike takes a little bit more preparation than a walk. You need to plan your route in advance and know exactly where you're going. I strongly recommend hiking with a companion—it's a lot more fun, anyway. If you haven't done much hiking or you're unfamiliar with an area, it makes sense to go out with a more experienced guide. At the very least, stop in at a ranger station and get some advice on good trails along with a trail map.

If you're unfamiliar with routes in your area or you don't have a partner, contact the local chapter of the Sierra Club or a local hiking club. Topographic maps, available at most outdoor stores and park headquarters, can save you from getting in over your head: A short hike can take all day if there are lots of ups and downs. Learn how to read elevation lines and look for switchbacks, which indicate steep terrain. Guidebooks take the guesswork out, with useful details about the length and difficulty of suggested hikes.

Always stay on the marked paths, and be aware of the trail signs and markers. Getting lost and getting caught by a sudden change in the weather are undoubtedly the most serious threats to your safety, but hiking in the backcountry has other hazards, ranging from plant irritants and ticks to unfriendly animals like bears and poisonous snakes. While poisonous plants are hard to avoid in some areas, run-ins with animals are rare, because most potentially harmful creatures are trying to get away from *you*. Before hiking, stop by the ranger station or check a guidebook to learn about local hazards.

Don't be put off by all these precautions: As long as you know where you're going and are prepared (see the checklist below), hiking is perfectly safe. It's a wonderful way to spend a day, whether you're in a nearby state park or off the beaten path at one of our spectacular national parks.

For a great walking vacation, many adventure travel companies feature mountain hiking trips in the U.S. and abroad. Some offer heli-hiking in which you're whisked to the top of a mountain range and set loose to wander; others have you hiking to a different country inn every day. These guided outings are ideal for both novices and experienced hikers.

What the Well-dressed Hiker Is Wearing

- High-top hiking boots with good traction. The high-top gives you ankle support for downhills and uneven ground. A deep tread pattern provides traction on loose or wet ground. Rocks along the trail can cause sore feet; a beefier sole offers more protection. You want plenty of room in the boot to accommodate thick socks. And watch your toes: If they're too close to the front of the boot, they'll get jammed on downhills.

- Thick socks, ideally polyester or a wool-poly blend, for blister prevention.
- A fanny pack or day pack.
- Lightweight long pants and a long-sleeved shirt will protect you from ticks, sun, and poisonous plants. Light colors reflect sunlight and show ticks (check for them periodically). Carry an extra layer of clothing and a waterproof jacket.
- Sunscreen, a hat, and sunglasses.
- Insect repellent.
- Plenty of water, and foods that pack well, like raisins, apples, and crackers.
- A pocketknife.
- Matches and a small flashlight, just in case you're out there longer than you expected.
- A topographic map, a guidebook, and a compass.
- Optional: A field guide to plants and birds; binoculars; camera.

WALKING CLUBS

I believe that one of the best ways to make something your own is to teach it to someone else. If you've mastered this walking program, you should be able to show another person how to do it. Demonstrating and explaining these techniques will really force you to get your ducks in a row.

Switching from student to teacher can revive your own excitement about walking, and it may turn out to be a life-changing experience for someone else. Maybe you have a friend or relative who could really use some regular exercise . . .

Along the same lines, why not start a walking club in your office or neighborhood? Aside from giving you the chance to share your knowledge, it's a great way to assemble a group of walking partners. It doesn't take much more than a few phone calls or hanging a sign on a bulletin board. You can organize lunchtime walks or weekend walks followed by a (low-fat) potluck supper.

You can get a pamphlet with advice on starting a walking club, including tips on recruiting and scheduling, from *Walking Magazine*'s Walking Club Alliance. Once you've established your club, you can join the Alliance. Then you'll receive a member kit that includes a leader's manual, a resource guide, and information on their awards program. For more information, write to the Walking Club Alliance, Walking, Inc., 9–11 Harcourt Street, Boston, MA 02116.

Maybe you're not the organizing type, but you'd like to join an existing walking club. You can find them in every state; some are race-walking oriented, but these usually welcome recreational walkers as well. There are also mall-walking clubs at most major shopping malls. A call to the mall management will usually produce a name of a walking group's organizer.

To find a walking club near you, send your name and address to *Walking Magazine*'s Walking Club Alliance coordinator, at the above address. You'll receive information on clubs in your area; if there is no existing club near you, you'll get tips on starting your own.

RACE WALKING

If you've really got the fast walking bug, and you're ready to go from walking for fitness to walking for sport, race walking is for you. WALKFIT will definitely give you a head start, by getting you in shape and teaching you some novice race-walking techniques, like the arm swing and foot action.

Race walking is mainly taught through race-walking clubs. These groups typically teach advanced techniques, train together, and participate in local and national track meets. You can get a listing of race-walking clubs by contacting *Walking Magazine*'s Walking Club Alliance, at the aforementioned address. Or contact the American Race-walking Association, P.O. Box 18325, Boulder, CO 80308, or the North American Racewalking Foundation, 1000 San Pasqual, #35, Pasadena, CA 91106.

ROAD RACES AND EVENTS

Whenever I travel, I keep an eye open for local road races. I love to go to these events, which are usually 5 or 10 kilometers in length, not to race but to go for a walk or a jog—usually on an especially nice, traffic-free route—with a bunch of fun people.

Last summer, during our vacation in Montana, Steve and I saw a notice for the Eagle Bend 5K and 10K Fun Run and Walk. We couldn't pass that up, so we turned out early on a Wednesday evening to join several dozen other folks who were walking and running along an absolutely beautiful route next to Flathead Lake in Bigfork. The emphasis was definitely on "fun," as each participant covered the course at his or her own pace. The first people across the finish line got a pat on the back, and when everyone was through, there was a random drawing for prizes. I even won a T-shirt!

If you've always imagined these events to be full of hard-core runners, elbowing for position from start to finish, take a closer look. While the people in the front of the pack may be racing, the majority of folks are there just to participate. Most local events now have large walking divisions. Sometimes you sign up specifically for a 5K walk, other times you just show up and walk the course. (Of course, if you're down to a 12-minute-per-mile walking pace, you might be faster than some of the joggers!)

In fact, in the last few years many road races have been transformed into something more like a big parade. These are community events, with people running and walking along, some pushing baby strollers or toting kids. Sometimes they're there for a cause, like fund-raising for a charity. Sometimes the cause is just to be outside on a beautiful day. At bigger events there are usually booths, with people giving away free samples or showing new fitness products. And at the end, of course, everybody gets a T-shirt.

Getting ready for an event can be great inspiration. If you know you're going to walk a 5K next month, you have an extra incentive to walk a little harder. A 5K event (3.1 miles) should be easily within your grasp once you've reached WALKFIT Level III (see Chapter 3). For walkers at Levels IV and V, finishing a 5K in 36 minutes or better is an excellent training goal.

INTERVAL WORKOUT

In Chapter 3, I talked about increasing the aerobic challenge of your walks with intervals: Alternating periods of high-intensity walking with slower recovery periods, so that your heart, lungs, and muscles work harder for short spurts than they could work continuously. Well, here's a workout that applies the same principle—interval training—in a slightly different way.

This interval workout is a way to put a little muscle in your walking workout. It consists of a series of "power moves," with "recovery" periods of walking in between. This is a fun workout—there's absolutely no boredom factor. It also develops lower-body strength and tones the buttocks and legs.

Training for a 10K

For a 10K (6.2 miles), you may want to do some extra distance training. Most walkers at Level IV or better should be able to walk six 15-minute miles: that's a 90-minute 10K. Six 12-minute miles (a 1:12 10K), however, is a real challenge. (Just for comparison, an elite race walker covers 10 kilometers in 40 to 45 minutes.)

If you are comfortable at a 12- or 13-minute mile pace, you can train to do a 1:15 10K. Here's how:

Keeping your pace close to 12 minutes per mile, gradually increase the length of your long walks. You don't want to increase distance by more than 10 percent per week, so if you're walking 3 miles now, you should add only a quarter-mile per week. Starting from 3 miles, you'd progress like this:

Week 1: 3.25
Week 2: 3.5
Week 3: 3.75
Week 4: 4.0
Week 5: 4.25
Week 6: 4.5

On race day, you should be able to complete a distance about one-third longer than your training walks, so you could probably do a 10K (6 miles) after six weeks of training.

With this kind of training, rest and recovery become more important. Limit your long, fast workouts to two to three per week. Alternate these with two easier days—slower or shorter—and a day or two of rest.

Start with a one-to-one ratio between the power moves and recovery periods: If you do 30 seconds worth of power moves, recover by walking for 30 seconds. As your fitness improves, increase the interval length, keeping the one-to-one ratio. When you get up to 90-second intervals, you can start reducing the recovery time. After a while, for example, you might be up to 90-second work intervals with 45 seconds of recovery in between.

These power moves are extremely demanding. You're probably ready for this workout when you are comfortable walking at a 13-minute-mile pace or better. Then it's important to start with small bites: Select an interval length that you can handle. You set yourself up for injury if you don't pace yourself.

THE WORKOUT

Start with a 10-minute walking warm-up in Foundation. Then begin your intervals:

Power Move #1: Pick Up the Pace

Speed up to a fast Workout pace. Don't go all out: It should feel like about 75 percent of full speed. To recover, slow down to an easy Workout pace (not Foundation). At the end of the rest interval, you should feel ready to go again.

Power Move #2: Side-Stepping

Move sideways, sliding your feet together but not crossing your legs. Lead with your right leg first, and recover by walking at a Workout pace. Then lead with your left leg and recover.

Power Move #3: Crossover Steps

Move sideways again, but this time allow your legs to cross. Your right leg first crosses in front of your left and then passes behind, so your hips are really swiveling. Go to your right, and then to your left, with recovery in between.

Power Move #4: Bounding

This is like taking giant, jumping steps. With each stride, you spring up as high as you can. You're jumping off your right leg, then your left leg, then your right leg, etc. Recover.

Power Move #5: Walking Backward

First check to make sure you've got a clear path (it helps to have a partner for this one). Then walk backward. Try to move quickly, but not so fast that you're likely to trip. Recover.

Finish with a 10-minute cool-down in Foundation.

With 30-second intervals, it will take you 14 minutes to go through all the moves once; with warm-up and cool-down, that's a 34-minute workout. If you have time, go through the power moves twice, for 28 minutes of intervals and a total workout time of 48 minutes.

WALK-JOG WORKOUTS

Another way to apply the interval concept is in a walk-jog workout. This workout is similar to the fast-walking intervals in Chapter 3, but instead of alternating two walking speeds, you'll alternate jogging and fast walking.

When you're walking fast, a slow jog makes for a great recovery interval, because you get to rest walking-specific muscles, like your shins and gluteals. Jogging feels like a release from really fast walking, and so the two paces complement one another, enabling you to keep going faster, longer.

This workout is a great way to add some variety to your training, and because it's a high-intensity workout, it's ideal on days when you don't have much time to exercise: 30 minutes of walk-jog intervals is a great speedy workout.

The jogging intervals are high-impact, so I recommend wearing running shoes for this one. Skip this workout if you have any orthopedic problems—knee, foot, back, or ankle problems—that are aggravated by running. I also don't recommend jogging if you're more than a little overweight, because the higher your weight, the greater the potential for problems from the high-impact portion of the workout.

Start with a Foundation warm-up for 5 to 10 minutes. For the walk/jog intervals, keep a one-to-one ratio between jogging and walking periods: a minute of jogging, followed by a minute of walking at a fast Workout pace. If you have trouble keeping that up, shorten the intervals, but keep the one-to-one ratio: Try 30 seconds of jogging, 30 seconds of walking.

As your fitness improves, you can make this workout more challenging in three ways: 1) Increase the length of your intervals in 15-second increments, eventually getting up to 2-minute intervals; 2) increase the duration of your workout; 3) increase your running and/or walking pace.

TREADMILLS

One of the things I love best about walking is that it gets me outdoors every day. Of course, I live in sunny southern California, where we don't have to worry about snowsuits and galoshes. If you live where the weather gets bad, a treadmill can be a lifesaver. If you don't belong to a health club, there are some very good treadmills available for in-home walking. While a good treadmill is not cheap, in certain climates it may be a worthwhile investment.

Treadmills have a few other advantages besides being weatherproof. With a treadmill, you always know your pace, and you can't cheat: The machine dictates the pace. In fact, a great way to learn to walk faster is to set the treadmill at a higher speed and force your feet to keep up. This approach is not without its hazards—if you crank it up too high you can go flying off the back—but you'd be amazed how much faster your feet can move on a treadmill than they can on the street.

Most treadmills also have a giving surface, which takes the low impact of walking and makes it almost nothing. Finally, if you've got kids to watch, over the course of a year a treadmill is probably cheaper than a babysitter.

Prices for a good treadmill range from about $500 to more than $2,000. With many of the high-priced models, you pay a lot for features like heart-rate monitors and workout programming capacity. If there's no room for fancy electronics in your budget, look for these important features in the less-expensive models: solid construction, a good motor, and adjustable speed and incline.

Most important is the motor that drives the belt. Cheap motors are noisy, and they don't last. This is especially true if larger people will be using the treadmill, since more weight means more work for the engine. Look for treadmills with at least 1.0 continuous-duty horsepower. Beware of claims like "1.0 peak horsepower."

You can tell a lot about a treadmill just by walking on it in the store. A good engine should hum quietly, even with a large person walking on it. The belt speed should be smooth and constant, with no hesitations or surges.

Check the speed range. If the treadmill isn't going to be used for running, you don't need a top speed above 8 MPH; if you'll be sharing it with a runner, you'll probably want one that goes up to 10 MPH. The speed adjustment is either a dial or a push button: Push-button control is more precise, but it's usually available only on machines that cost over $1,000. If you're looking at a machine with a dial, or rheostat, check it out carefully in the store: How quickly does the belt respond when you move the dial? Is it hard to set it to a precise speed?

You can adjust the incline on most treadmills; most go up to a 10 to 15 percent grade, which is plenty. On less expensive models, you have to get off the machine and set the incline manually. Automatic incline adds several hundred dollars to the price tag.

One last word of advice before you try to find space in your home for a treadmill: Like most exercise equipment, a poorly made treadmill is probably worse than no tread-mill at all. Compare the price of a "cheap" treadmill to a health club membership before you bring home next spring's garage sale centerpiece.

WALKING VIDEOTAPES

Before you invest in a treadmill, you might want to look into another, less expensive option for in-home walking workouts: walking-based exercise videotapes. These tapes are similar to other exercise videos, but they're based on walking movements or steps, instead of dance aerobics. There are a number of indoor-walking workouts available at video stores; mine is called "March to Fitness."

8

‗

WALKFIT
Stretches

Stretching is a lot like flossing your teeth: It seems like such a minor thing that you're tempted to skip it, but it can actually save you a lot of pain in the long run. When you stretch, you increase the range of motion in your muscles and joints, which is another way of saying it helps you move more freely. That makes it easier to master certain fast-walking techniques, like hip rotation and leg extension. So stretching can improve your speed.

Stretching also relieves excess muscle tension, which makes your body feel better and may reduce the chance of muscle cramps or injury. One of the first signs of aging is that our tissues, including muscles, tendons, and ligaments, become less elastic—they have less give. Your flexibility starts to decline in your 20s, so it's important to stretch, in order to prevent muscle pulls or tendinitis (inflammation of the tendons).

Stretching is more of an art than a science. There's no universally agreed-upon right or wrong way to do it. Let your muscles be your guide: If you feel a mild tension in a muscle you're stretching, you're doing something right; if you don't feel anything or if it hurts, you're probably doing something wrong.

WHEN TO STRETCH

When is the best time to stretch? It's a question that exercise experts disagree on. After years of experimenting with stretching before, during, and after workouts, I've come to the conclusion that it's a matter of what works best for you. Here are some guidelines. Experiment with them, and see what makes your body feel best.

• Stretch *lightly* before your walk. Many fitness professionals advise against stretching before you've warmed up, because you're pulling on cold, tight muscles. But no one has ever proven that people who stretch before exercise get more injuries, and many people find that they feel better when they stretch problem areas *gently* and *gradually* before starting to exercise.

• I prefer to warm up those tight spots after walking for five to eight minutes. I don't do a full-body stretch at that point, but I spend a minute or two loosening up trouble spots, like my shoulders, neck, and shins.

• The best time for a deep, full-body stretch is right after your walk, when your muscles are still loose. This is when I work on anything that feels tight, and I stretch everything else just to make sure.

• Think about stretching at other times, as well, like first thing in the morning, in front of the TV, or as a break from sitting at a desk.

STRETCHING TIPS

- Hold each stretch for about 20 seconds.
- Stretch to the point of mild tension, but not pain. As the muscle relaxes, you can gently increase the stretch.
- For problem areas, repeat the stretch.
- Breathe naturally while you stretch.
- Always use slow, controlled movements. Don't bounce or bob.

THE STRETCHES

This set of stretches is designed specifically to complement your WALKFIT workout. If you do all 14 exercises, you'll get a great, full-body stretch, with special concentration on areas that tend to get tight during fast walking—the shins, neck, and shoulders. It will take you only about five minutes to do them all, but if a particular stretch doesn't seem to do much for you, skip it. If you've got no patience at all for stretching, at least take a minute to stretch any muscles that are particularly tight.

These are suggested body positions, to use as a guide. Your body is unique, and you may find that you get a deeper or more comfortable stretch by modifying the illustrated positions. Or, if you don't feel a stretch where you're supposed to, modify the position, slowly and gently, until you do.

Calves (gastrocnemius and soleus muscle groups, Achilles tendon)

A. Take a giant step forward with your left foot. With your left leg bent and your right leg straight, move your hips forward. Keep both feet pointing forward, and keep your right heel on the ground. You should feel the stretch in your right calf. Repeat with your right foot forward.

B. (Not shown.) Use the same position as above, but this time lower your hips slightly as you bend your back leg at the knee. Now you should feel the stretch slightly lower and deeper in your calf. Repeat with the other leg.

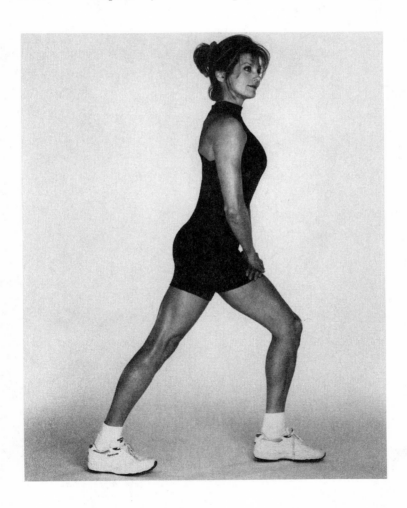

Front of the Thigh (quadriceps)

Stand near something you can hang onto for balance—a wall, pole, or chair. Grasp your right foot with your right hand, steadying yourself with your left hand. Ease your foot toward your buttocks. Keep your knees together and your hips facing forward and square, not rotated. Repeat with the other leg.

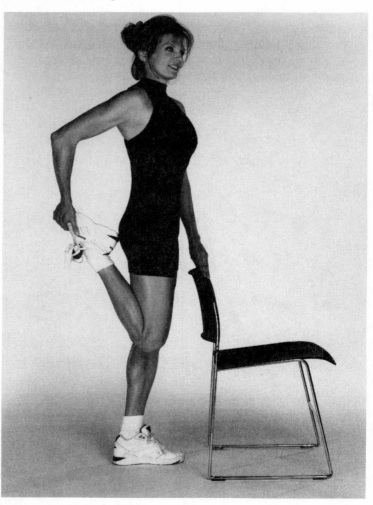

Back of the Thigh (hamstrings)

Raise your right leg and rest it on an elevated platform: a park bench or a car bumper. (It doesn't have to be high—just a foot or two off the ground). Straighten your right leg. With a slight bend in your left leg, and your hips square to your extended leg, bend forward from the hips—not from the waist. If you do it correctly, you shouldn't have to tilt your upper body very far forward before you feel the stretch in the back of your leg. Repeat with your left leg extended.

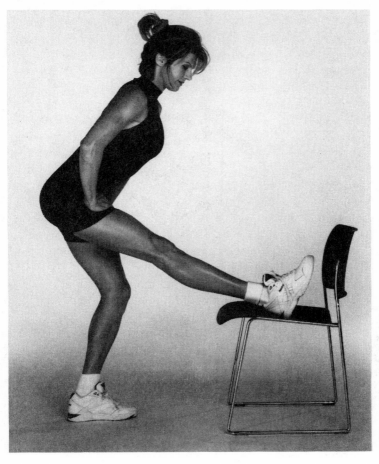

Inner Thigh (adductors)

Sit on the floor and bring the soles of your feet together. Now bring your feet in as close to your buttocks as you can. Use your elbows to push your knees toward the floor. You should feel the stretch on the inside of your thighs.

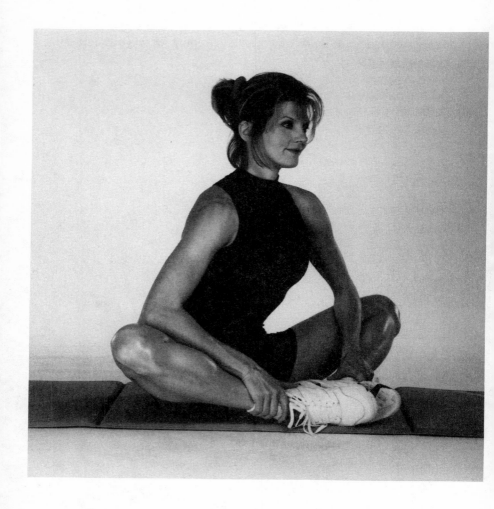

Hips and Buttocks (gluteals)

Lying on your back, use your left hand to pull your right knee across your body and toward the ground on your left side. Keep your right shoulder flat on the ground, with your arm outstretched. By slightly altering where you place your bent leg, you'll feel the stretch in different parts of your hips and buttocks. Try moving your knee toward your head, then away from it. Repeat with the other leg.

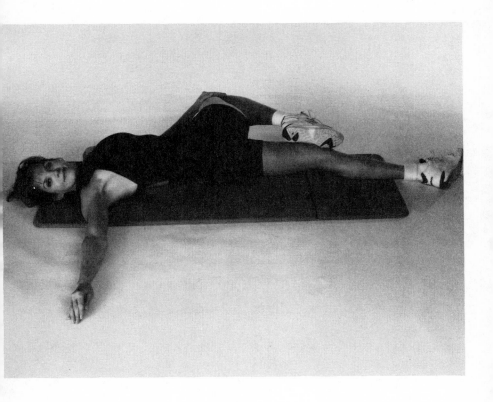

Lower Back

Kneel on all fours, with your hands and knees spread evenly, and your neck relaxed. Contract your abdominals, drop your head, and round your back up, like a cat. Hold, then return to a flat back position.

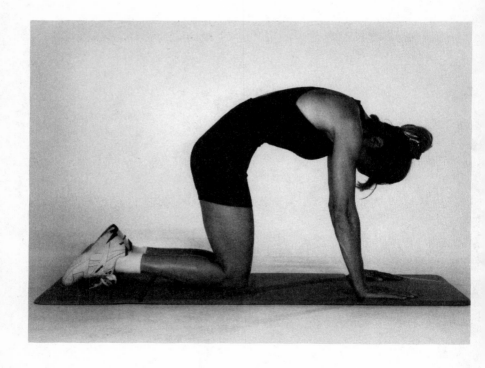

Hip Flexor

Your right leg is bent 90 degrees at the knee, and your left leg is straight behind you, with your toes extended. Place your hands on the floor, one hand on each side of your right leg, and press your hips toward the floor. You should feel the stretch in the front of the left hip. Repeat with your right leg back.

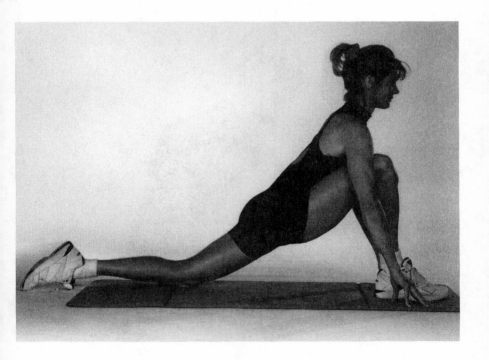

Side Stretch

Stand with your feet shoulder-width apart, your knees bent slightly, and your toes pointing straight ahead. Place your right hand on your hip while you extend your left arm above your head. Slowly bend at the waist to the right, and hold. Repeat to the other side.

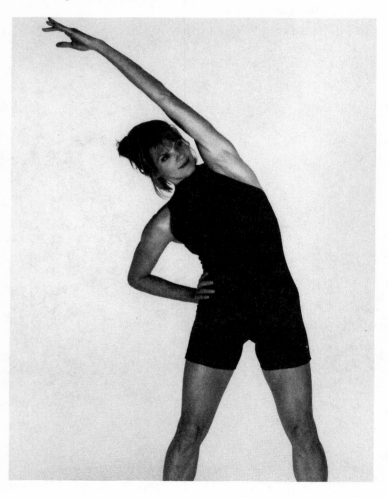

Shoulders

Stand with your knees slightly bent. Raise your right arm in front of you, to shoulder height. Grasp your right upper arm with your left hand, and pull your right arm across your body. You should feel the stretch in your shoulder and upper arm. By moving your shoulder up toward your ears and then down, you'll feel the stretch in slightly different places. Repeat with the left arm.

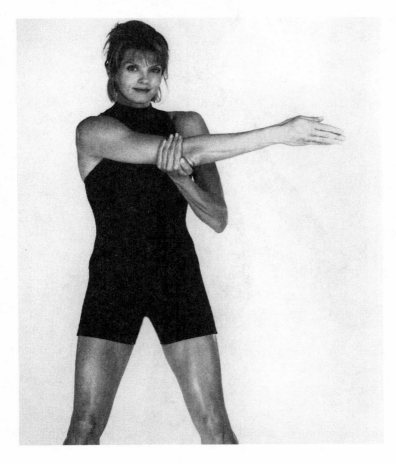

Chest

Stand with your feet shoulder-width apart, your knees bent slightly, and your toes pointing straight ahead. Clasp your hands behind your back. Slowly straighten your arms, then lift your hands and your chest. You should feel your chest expanding, and you'll feel a stretch in your shoulders, too.

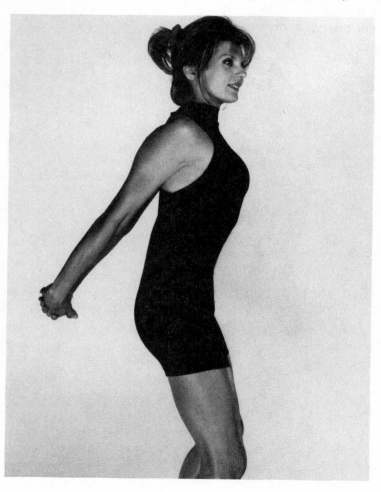

Upper Back (latissimus dorsi)

Stand with your feet shoulder-width apart, your knees bent slightly, and your toes pointing straight ahead. Reach forward with both arms and grasp your left wrist with your right hand. Now round your back and hollow out your stomach—as if you got punched in the gut. Without rotating your upper body, pull your left arm out and across to the right side of your body. Feel the stretch along the back of your left arm and the left side of your upper back. Repeat, stretching your right side.

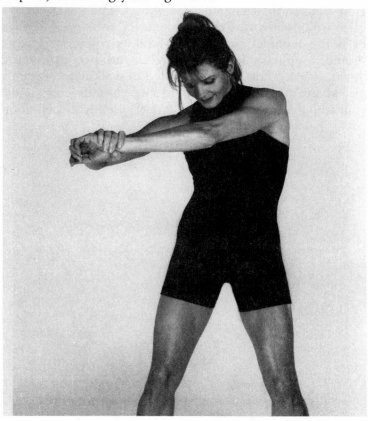

Neck

A. Stand with your feet shoulder-width apart, your knees bent slightly, and your toes pointing straight ahead. Drop your head forward, stretching the muscles in the back of your neck. Bring your head back up. Now place your hands behind your back, and grab your right wrist with your left hand. Drop your head to your left shoulder, and at the same time pull down on your right arm, to stretch the neck from both ends. Bring your head back up, and then repeat to the other side: Pull down on your left arm as you drop your head to the right side.

B. (Not shown.) Relax the base of your neck further by doing shoulder shrugs and shoulder rolls. Bring your shoulders up to your ears, then relax and drop them back down. (I like to do this one while I'm walking, to remind me where my shoulders should and shouldn't be.) Roll your shoulders, making four circles forward, then four circles backward.

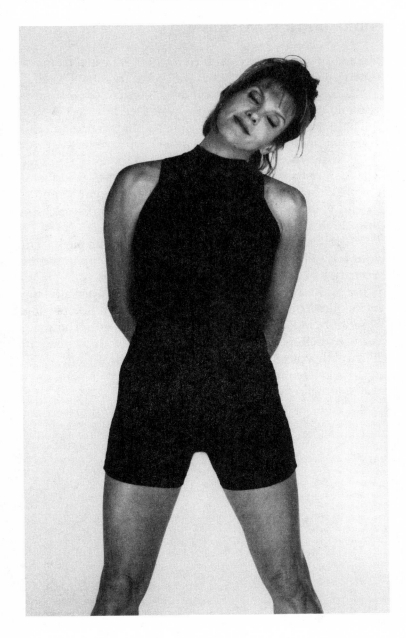

Shins (anterior tibialis)

Here are a couple of great shin stretches I learned from six-time national champion race walker Maryanne Torrellas.

A. Sit on the floor, with your legs extended in front of you and your toes pointing upward. Place a towel around the ball of your right foot, holding the ends of the towel in your hands. Push against the towel with your foot, and resist with your hands so that your foot doesn't move. This contracts the shin muscles. Hold this position for 15 seconds, then relax for 2 seconds. Then use your hand to extend your foot completely (toes pointed), to stretch the shin. Repeat with your left foot.

B. (Not shown.) You can also lie on your back, with your left foot on the floor and your right foot up in the air. Your right knee is bent slightly. Imagine that your big toe is the tip of a pen, and try to draw the uppercase alphabet in the air. Your foot will move through a complete range of motion, loosening up your shins. At first, your shins may get tired before you get to Z, so just go as far as you can. Eventually you should be able to make it through the entire alphabet. Repeat with your left foot.

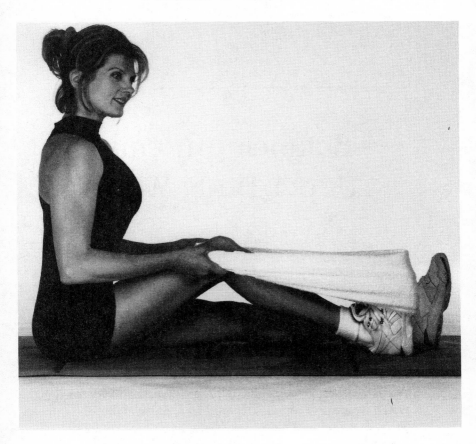

9

Balancing It Out: Upper-Body Work

Walking, like most aerobic exercise, is lower-body driven. That's because moving the big muscles in the legs is the best way to make your heart and lungs work. When you walk, your legs support the weight of your body, and they encounter resistance from the ground. This strengthens the muscles of the leg.

While a vigorous arm swing increases the cardiovascular demands of walking and increases your calorie burning, it's not really effective training for your upper body. Since your arms aren't working against any resistance, they don't get stronger. Some people try to remedy this inequity by carrying hand weights while walking, but I don't recommend walking with weights.

Why not? Because even if you do carry hand weights, you're *still* not getting a great upper-body workout. So why compromise the quality of your walks with hand weights?

When I see people carrying weights, they've usually got their arms hanging at their sides. The weights aren't doing them any good hanging there, and they've sacrificed the cardiovascular benefits of a vigorous arm swing. If you do pump your arms with weights in your hands, the extra mass can exaggerate your natural motion. Since your arms and legs need to work together, that can throw off your whole stride.

If total body fitness is what you're after, I recommend supplementing your walking program with upper-body strength training. This can be done in an exercise class or a weight room, or you can use the program in this chapter. With these exercises, in just two 30-minute sessions per week you'll strengthen and tone the muscles in your arms, back, and abdominals.

BENEFITS OF STRENGTH TRAINING

When it comes to toning or building muscle, strength training is the way to go. Maintaining your muscles is important, and not just because a toned body looks good: Lean muscle tissue burns more calories than fat tissue. By keeping your lean muscle mass high, you increase your metabolism—the number of calories you burn on a daily basis. That helps with weight control.

Keeping your muscles in good shape also helps you in daily life, with everything from walking the dog to carrying newspapers out for recycling. Finally, increased upper-body strength can help increase your walking speed, because a stronger arm swing will generate more momentum.

WORKOUT GUIDELINES

You'll need a thick pillow, a chair, and two sets of light dumbbells (1 and 3 pounds for beginners, 3 and 5 pounds for intermediate and advanced). I've made recommendations about which weight (light or heavy) you should use for each exercise, but you can substitute the other one if it feels better:

- These strength-training exercises should be done a minimum of twice a week. It should take 30 to 40 minutes to complete them. Always allow at least 36 hours rest between strength-training sessions.
- Start with five or ten minutes of Foundation walking to increase your circulation and warm up your muscles. Walk around the block, walk in place, or walk up and down the stairs. As you're walking, do some shrugs and some large circular motions with your arms to get your upper body loosened up as well.
- Do each exercise in a slow, controlled, manner. Don't let momentum move the weight for you.
- Control both directions of the movement. It's not lifting and dropping.
- Move the weight through the full range of motion that the directions indicate. Raise it all the way up, and lower it all the way back down.
- Breathe normally as you work your muscles. Don't hold your breath.
- You want to feel the muscle group you're working. If you don't feel it contracting, you're either doing the exercise incorrectly or not using enough weight.
- Start with 2 sets of 8 repetitions of each exercise, and gradually build up to 12 repetitions. (If you can't maintain good form and complete a set of 8 repetitions, use less weight.) Rest for only 30 seconds to a minute between sets.
- When you can comfortably do 2 sets of 12 repetitions, you're ready for more weight. When you increase the weight, start with 2 sets of 8 repetitions, and work your way back up to 2 sets of 12 repetitions. With

strength training, as with walking and all exercise, you need to keep challenging your body if you want continued results.
• Finish the workout with the upper-body stretches in Chapter 8.

THE EXERCISES

THE CHEST (PECTORALIS)

Push-ups

Place your hands on the ground, slightly wider than your shoulders. If you're strong enough, support your weight with your hands and your toes. If not, support yourself with your hands and your knees.

Keeping your abdominals tight and your back rigid, lower yourself until your chest touches the floor. Your elbows should make about a 45-degree angle with your sides.

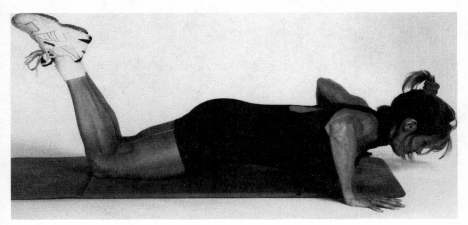

Flys (light dumbbells)

Lie on your back on the pillow, with your legs up. Extend your arms over your head, with the weights in your hands. Your palms should be facing each other, with your elbows bent slightly.

Now lower the weights to just above shoulder level, keeping that slight bend in your elbows. Your palms should be facing straight up. As you bring the weight back up, rotate your arms so that when the weights come together, your pinkie fingers are together. Rotate them again as you lower the weight, so that your palms are facing up again at the bottom of the move. Keep the bend in your elbow at all times, and feel the chest muscles working as you lift and lower.

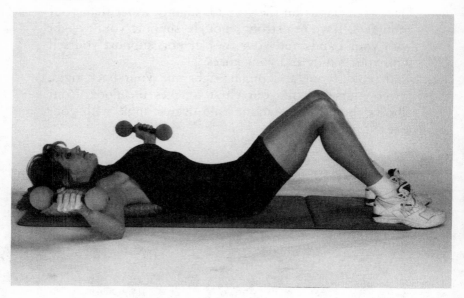

UPPER ARMS (TRICEPS)

French Press (heavy dumbbell)

Stand with a slight bend in your knees. Holding a heavy weight with both hands, extend your arms above your head. Keeping your upper arms next to your head, bend your elbows and lower the weight all the way back toward your shoulders. Then extend your elbows and lift the weight back up over your head. Your upper arms should stay next to your ears—don't let your elbows drift out to the side. You should feel the muscles in the back of your upper arm working.

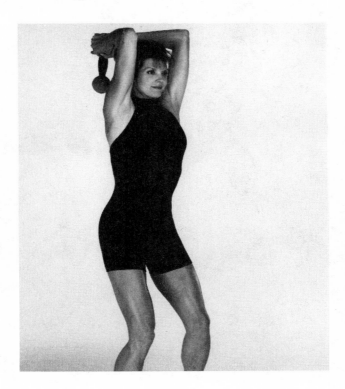

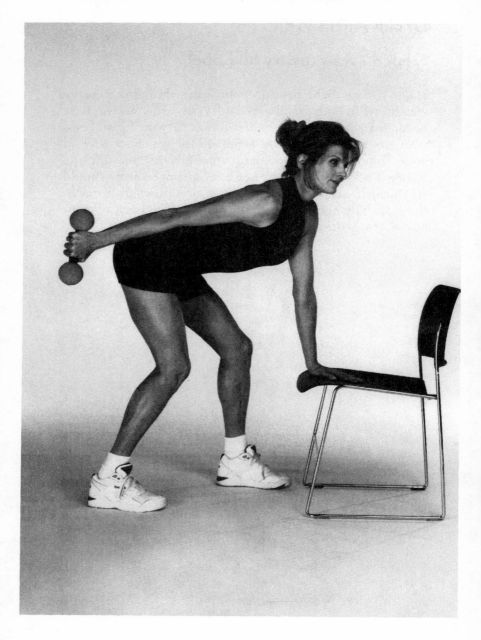

Triceps Kick-Back (light dumbbell)

Lean forward from the waist, supporting yourself with your left hand on the chair. Your upper body should be parallel to the floor, and your legs should be slightly bent. Bend your right arm, with your elbow along your side. Your right forearm should be hanging down, with the dumbbell in your hand and your palm facing in toward your body.

Now straighten your arm back behind you, and rotate the weight so your palm faces up at the end of the movement. Rotate again as you lower the weight, so your palm faces your body again at the end of the movement. Your elbow should stay by your side as you lift and lower the weight. Repeat with your left arm.

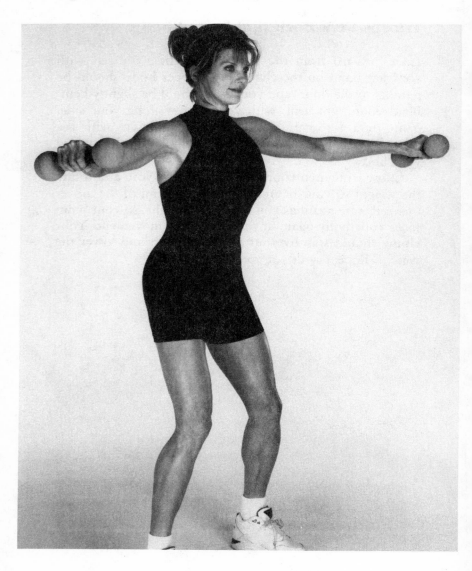

SHOULDERS (DELTOIDS)

Each shoulder muscle is actually a group of three muscle segments. It takes three exercises to work them all.

Side Raises (heavy dumbbells)

Stand, holding the dumbbells at your sides, with your palms facing in. Keep a slight bend in your knees. Lift the weights up and to the side, to shoulder level. Keep your palms facing down, and don't raise the weights above your shoulders. Your elbows should be slightly bent, not locked out.

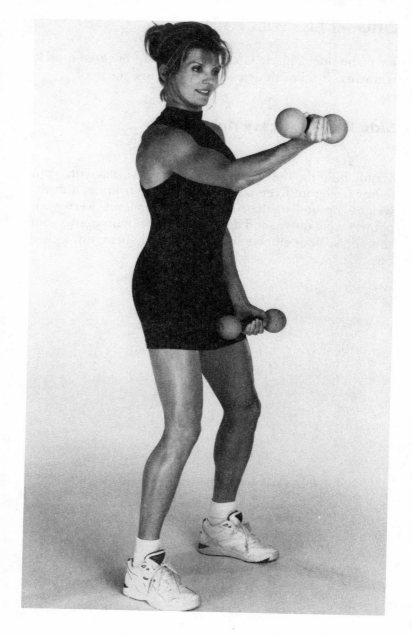

Front Raises (heavy dumbbells)

Start in the same position as for side raises, but with your palms facing forward. Lift one arm at a time, alternating left and right, and lift the weight forward and out slightly. Keep your palms up and elbows down throughout the movement. Maintain a slight bend in your elbows, and be careful not to arch your lower back to heave or fling the weight up.

Rear Raises (light dumbbells)

Sit on the edge of the chair, with the dumbbells on the floor in front of you. Bend forward, resting your upper body on the pillow for support. Pick up the dumbbells with your palms facing in. Now lift the weight up and out to the side, keeping a slight bend in your elbows; it's like flapping your wings. At the top of the movement, the weight should be straight out from your shoulders, not back at your waist, and your shoulders, elbows, and palms should be at the same level.

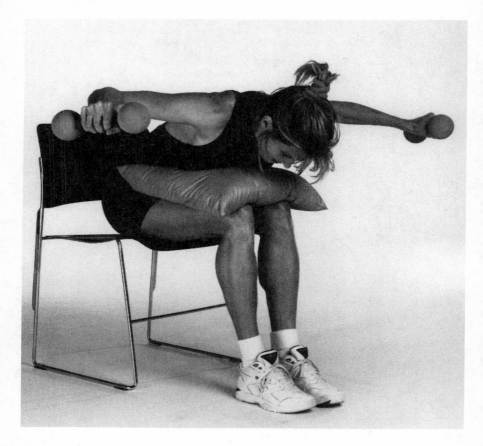

UPPER BACK

One-arm Row (heavy dumbells)

Bend over, supporting yourself with the chair. Your upper body should be roughly parallel to the floor. Stand with your left foot forward, your right foot back, and your knees bent slightly. Your right arm is hanging straight down, with both heavy dumbbells in your hand (this is a big, strong muscle group). At the beginning of the move, you should feel your back stretching, and your shoulder blades should be as far apart as possible.

Now lift the weights until your upper arm and elbow reach the level of your back—no higher. As you lift, think about bringing your shoulder blades together. You should feel this in your back, not your arm or shoulder. Keep your upper arm relaxed throughout the movement.

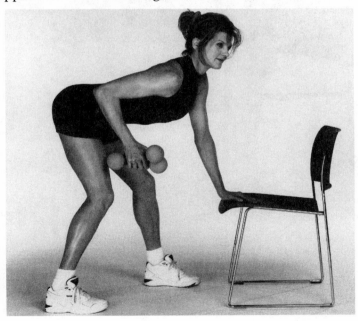

Shrugs (heavy dumbbells)

Sit on the edge of the chair, with the dumbbells on the floor next to your feet. Bend forward, resting your upper body on your pillow for support. Pick up the dumbbells, and hold them with your palms facing in. Lift the weights by shrugging, or drawing your shoulder blades together. Don't lift out with your arms. Try to keep your neck relaxed as you do this one.

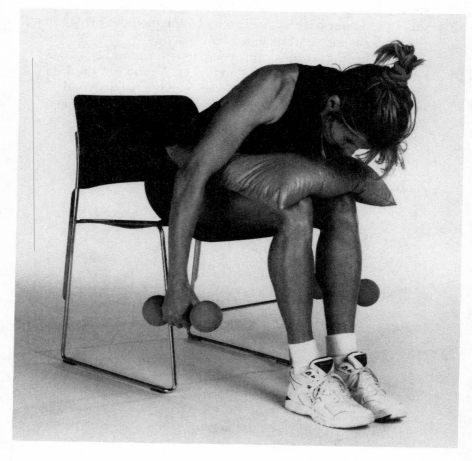

BICEPS

Straight Dumbbell Curls (heavy dumbbells)

Stand with your knees bent slightly and your arms extended at your sides. The dumbbells are in your hands and your palms are facing forward. Keeping your elbows at your side, curl the weight up to shoulder level, allowing your elbows to move forward just an inch or two. Stop the upward movement before your forearms are pointed straight up, then lower the weight back down.

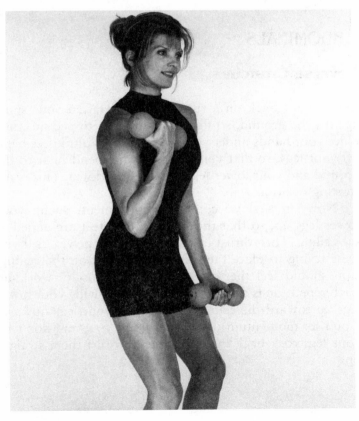

Supinated Dumbbell Curls (heavy dumbbells)

(Not shown.) Start in the same position as for the straight dumbbell curls, except that your palms are facing in, toward your thighs. Rotate your forearms as you raise the weight, so that at the end of the movement your palms are facing your shoulders. Rotate them again as you lower the weight back to the starting position. Again, keep your elbows at your sides, allowing them to move forward just an inch or two as you curl your arm up.

ABDOMINALS

Reverse Crunches

Lie on your back on a rug or carpet. Flatten your spine against the ground, so that your pelvis is tipped up, then place your hands under your pelvis. With your knees bent, lift your legs, so that your thighs are perpendicular to the ground and your lower legs are hanging down. This is the starting position.

Now, in a slow, controlled movement, swing your lower legs up, so that the soles of your feet are aimed at the ceiling. Then thrust upward from your pelvis, as if you were trying to place the soles of your feet on the ceiling. You should feel the lower abdominal muscles working. Each repetition is a two-part movement: Swing your lower legs up toward the ceiling, then thrust your legs upward. Don't let momentum do the work for you, and don't let your legs rock back over your head; thrust them straight up.

Now Steve and I *make* time to walk together, even if it means getting a babysitter. As I developed WALKFIT, Steve would join me for walks. Sure, he'd whine about his shins hurting sometimes, but it was always great to have him along, and his feedback helped make the program better.

Walking *is* great exercise, but it's much, much more than that. I've read an awful lot about the benefits of walking—the cardiovascular benefits and musculo-skeletal benefits and psychological benefits. I don't think I've ever read that walking is one of the best ways to nurture a relationship, but it is.

STEP ONTO THAT ROAD

There are so many good reasons to walk, just as there are so many good reasons to eat right. This book contains what I believe to be a very realistic, effective strategy for making healthy, lasting changes to your lifestyle. The rest is up to you.

As you set off in this new, healthy direction, keep in mind that it is your body, with all its strengths and flaws, that must carry you. Let walking be a way to get comfortable with the body you have, to become aware of how it works for you, and to make it work even better.

Now, step off onto that new road, and see just how far your body can take you.

really new roads; they were just detours. Eventually she would "quit" the diet, revert to old habits, and gain back what she'd lost.

In 1992 Connie decided to try again. This time, she turned to WALKFIT and the low-fat diet outlined in Chapter 5. Her goal was to lose 102 pounds and keep it off for one year—not an easy thing to do.

"You set goals and you're never sure if you're going to reach them," Connie said to me when we met in San Francisco. "But if you make the decision that you want to change your life, and you start out slowly, and you make yourself do it, you get results."

Connie gradually worked up to 1 mile of walking a day, and her weight began to drop. After nine months, she was up to 4 miles of walking and down to 160 pounds. In the same time, her blood pressure dropped from a dangerous 160/102 to below normal, at 112/50, and her cholesterol dipped 80 points, to well below normal.

A year after heading off in a new direction, Connie feels confident that this is a lasting change. "I have no desire to eat the way I used to—I feel too good now," she says. "The way I'm eating and exercising is sensible. It's something I know I can do for the rest of my life."

Connie Harris made a change. She walked away from tiredness, from dizziness and high blood pressure, from aches in her back, feet, and legs. She walked away from having no self-esteem and being embarrassed to be seen by her friends. "You can only do it when you're ready to do it for *yourself*," Connie says now. "When you're tired of the way you are."

When you set off on a new road, you can't know exactly where you'll end up. As Connie said, you can never be sure of reaching your goals, but you can also never anticipate all the wonderful things that can happen, either.

Every evening, when Connie sets out for her walk, she's joined by her husband, Randy, an Air Force recruiter. Connie's good habit has become their shared good habit, and an opportunity to spend important time together every day.

Randy told me that walking "saved Connie's life and our marriage of eighteen years," and Connie agrees. "When I weighed 237 pounds, I was miserable, and that reflects on other parts of your life. We were neither one of us happy with each other or with ourselves," she says. "We're so much closer now. We've been married for eighteen years, and now it's like we've been married three years again, because I'm more like the person I used to be."

WALKING THE DOG

Walking has had some of the same positive affects on my marriage. Steve and I walked together when I was pregnant with Katie, and then again when I was expecting Perrie. Walking gave us a time when we could both relax and enjoy one another's company. It drew us closer.

After Perrie was born, things changed. Now we had two kids and we were both busy with our careers. There was no chance to talk anymore. It wasn't that we loved one another any less, but we came home in the evening, and after playing with the girls and reading to them, we didn't have a whole lot of energy left for one another.

Then, last year, Steve brought home a puppy for the girls, despite my protests. I figured the *last* thing we needed around our house was this furry tornado with four legs and a tail. But Jessie the chocolate Lab came with an advantage that I never would have guessed: We had to walk him.

Steve and the girls and I started walking the dog around the neighborhood every night. It didn't take long for both Steve and me to realize how much we'd missed walking together. It was so good to be on common ground again, to be back in this peaceful environment in which we could talk and make one another laugh.

10

A New Direction

Each of us has the right and the responsibility to assess the roads which lie ahead, and those over which we have traveled, and if the future road looms ominous or unpromising, and the roads back uninviting, then we need to gather our resolve and, carrying only the necessary baggage, step off that road into another direction. If the new choice is also unpalatable, without embarrassment, we must be ready to change that as well.

—Maya Angelou, "Wouldn't Take Nothing
for My Journey Now"

On a recent trip to New York, I was browsing in a bookstore when I happened upon a collection of essays by Maya Angelou. I bought the book, and when I sat down to read it I came across this passage. I was completely stunned: It was as if this remarkable woman was speaking my mind. Here she was, eloquently making the exact point that I'd been struggling for weeks to put into words.

I want to leave you with this message: It's time to gather your resolve and step off into another direction.

Walking and eating well are two important ways in which we can take care of ourselves. These actions make us more alive, by improving our health and vitality. They give us pleasure and enhance our sense of ourselves. I think you picked up this book in part because you know that.

You may also have turned to this book because the road back is uninviting. You've had enough of neglecting yourself. You're tired of having no energy, tired of hating your body, tired of feeling guilty about what you eat. You don't want to be limited by your weight anymore. You're sick of thinking, "I really should get more exercise."

Or maybe you've assessed the road ahead, and it's looking a little ominous. You can imagine how you'll feel in five years if you don't do something now. You know that heart disease or diabetes or hypertension runs in your family, and that your lifestyle will make you sick. You can see, when you look at people you love, what life will be like in 20 years if you don't start taking care of yourself.

There may be other ways in which your life needs changing, issues that you need to address that are more complicated and perhaps more important than diet and exercise. But this is a place to start. The road to wellness is easy to find: I'm even giving you a detailed map.

All you have to do is get started. Don't be daunted by how long the journey looks or by its steepness. If it's all you can manage, start by walking for just 20 minutes, three times a week. It's a beginning.

You have a right to be healthy and to live comfortably in your body. You have a responsibility to yourself, and to the people you love, to take these important, life-affirming steps.

"I CAN DO THIS FOR THE REST OF MY LIFE"

Back in Chapter 2, I introduced you to Connie Harris, the nurse from New York State who changed her life dramatically with walking and healthy eating.

Connie, who weighed 237 pounds, had tried all kinds of crash diets; she'd once lost 60 pounds in four months by "jogging and starving herself." But these diets weren't

Cross-Knee Crunches

Lie on your back on the floor with your feet on the floor. Place your left hand behind your head, and extend your right arm out to the side. Curl up, bringing your left shoulder and elbow across your body toward your right knee. You should feel this one working the muscles in your sides: the obliques. Repeat, bringing your right shoulder and elbow together with your left leg.

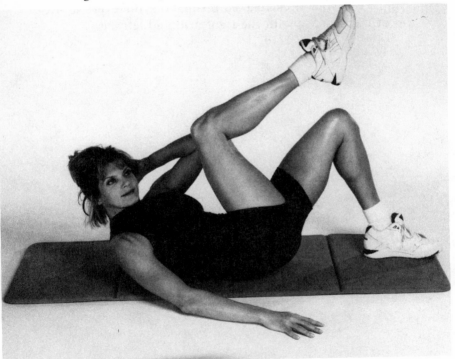

LOWER BACK (SPINAL ERECTORS)

Hyperextensions

Lie on your stomach on the floor, supported by your pillow, with your arms in front of you, like Superman. Now raise your left arm and right leg about a foot off the floor, then lower them back down to the ground. Lift and lower your arm and leg with a slow, controlled motion—no jerking. Keep your neck relaxed throughout the exercise. Repeat the exercise with the right arm and left leg.

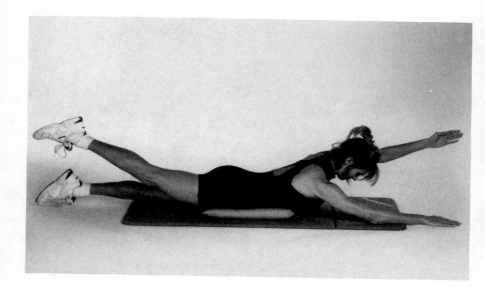

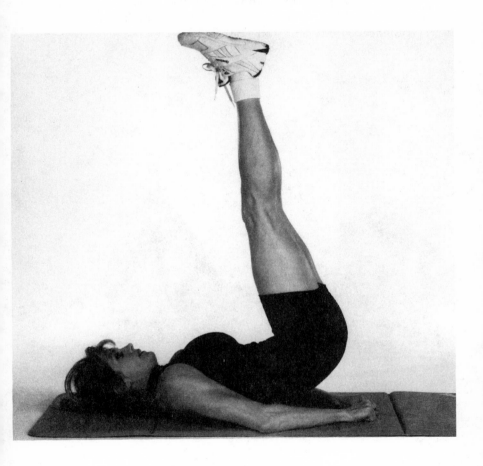

Crunches

Lie on your back on the floor with your feet on the floor and your hands behind your head. Curl up, bringing your upper back off the ground. When you're doing it right, you should feel your abdominal muscles contracting—not your neck, back, or leg muscles. Use your hands to support your head, but don't pull your head up.

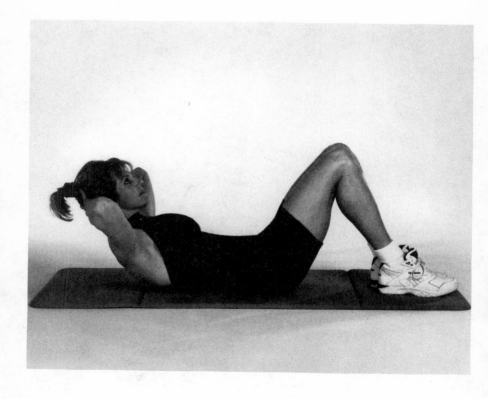